WEIGHT!
A Better Way to Lose
Winning the Battle Through Spiritual Motivation

Roger F. Campbell
Third Edition

kregel
PUBLICATIONS

Grand Rapids, MI 49501

Weight! A Better Way to Lose: Winning the Battle Through Spiritual Motivation, third edition

Copyright © 1976, 1988, 1999 by Roger F. Campbell

Published by Kregel Publications, a division of Kregel, Inc., P.O. Box 2607, Grand Rapids, MI 49501. Kregel Publications provides trusted, biblical publications for Christian growth and service. Your comments and suggestions are valued.

For more information about Kregel Publications, visit our web site at www.kregel.com

Cover and book design: Frank Gutbrod

Library of Congress Cataloging-in-Publication Data
Campbell, Roger F.
  Weight! A better way to lose: winning the battle through spiritual motivation / by Roger F. Campbell.
    p.   cm.
  Includes bibliographical references.
  1. Weight loss—Religious aspects—Christianity.
I. Title.
RM222.2.C2753   1998   613.2'5—dc 21   98-44657
                                                              CIP

ISBN 0-8254-2349-x

Printed in the United States of America

1 2 3 4 5 / 03 02 01 00 99

To Pauline
Whose example and research
made this book possible

Contents

Preface

"Thank you for caring!"

That expression of appreciaton came from a woman who had attended my first weight control class some twenty years ago. Her response to my presentation of a Christian approach to becoming thin and trim alerted me to the need of bringing hope to the great number of hurting people who struggle with the problem of being overweight.

The name given that first series of classes on weight control was *Lose Weight the Bible Way*. When Victor Books published the program in a book, we called it *Weight! A Better Way to Lose*. And many have found that title to be a true expression of experience.

Some have said that studying *Weight! A Better Way to Lose* has enabled them to adopt a lifestyle that has brought benefits well beyond weight control. Recently, a man called to say he thought the title should be *A Better Way to Live*.

Thin, Trim, and Triumphant enlarges upon the original plan and shares new insights. This book includes a number of personal testimonies from those who have been successful in losing weight by translating the concepts of *Weight! A Better Way to Lose* into their lives.

This new book contains all the principles found in the first one and adds a considerable amount of information that should make it even more helpful. The questions at the end of each chapter are intended to aid you in understanding and retaining the material presented. They also make the book more usable for group study.

I expect *Thin, Trim, and Triumphant* to help you achieve the proper weight for you. But I also expect this book to help you overcome in many areas of life.

Thin, Trim, and Triumphant says nothing about fasting. (Though the Bible contains a considerable amount of information on fasting, none of it relates to weight control.) Instead, this book is about a satisfying lifestyle with which you can be content to live for the rest of your life.

If you want to lose twenty pounds in the next ten days, my plan is not for you. Close the book. On the other hand, if you are fed up with fad diets that have kept you losing one week and gaining the next, you may be ready for a permanent solution to your problem. You may be ready to change to a Bible-centered lifestyle that can make it possible for you to become thin, trim, and triumphant.

1

Does God Really Care?

If you're down today because your weight is up, you are not alone. Unfortunately, the mood swings of many overweight people are controlled by the ups and downs of their bathroom scales.

Millions of hurting people in this weight-conscious world are pursuing some kind of diet or exercise plan, fighting the battle of the bulge. This passion to scale down has not gone unnoticed. The cry for success in weight control has given birth to a publishing bonanza and a weight-loss business boom.

Articles about weight loss are regular fare in most major magazines, and uncounted books have been written on the subject, many of them becoming bestsellers. Weight loss and exercise classes are multiplying, as are reducing resorts. And the public appetite for this kind of information and help seems insatiable.

Perhaps you've tried some of these programs in an effort to solve your weight problem. You may have even enjoyed temporary success. Then, because you did not make a permanent lifestyle change, those unwanted pounds returned, causing you to be more discouraged than ever.

Does the Bible Have the Answer?

Here you are opening a book about achieving weight control through applying principles of living found in the Bible. And this raises an important question: Does God really care about your weight problem?

Some think not.

While being interviewed on a call in radio talk show, I was scolded soundly by a listener who called to complain about my biblical approach to weight control. She accused me of using valuable time and effort to teach biblical concepts on a subject in which God has no interest.

At one time, I would have agreed with this angry caller. I had been in the ministry for nearly twenty years before realizing that a sizeable segment of my congregation was struggling with a serious problem that I had thought to be unrelated to biblical truth. I knew that alcoholics could be made sober; drug addicts could be delivered; those tempted to immorality could gain strength to overcome their temptations. But it never occurred to me that God might be concerned about people being overweight.

Now I know that I was wrong.

God cares about all of our needs.

Anything that troubles us concerns our Lord, including matters of health and appearance. His love provides this kind of all-encompassing interest in our deepest and most personal needs ... because that's what love is all about.

The Circle of God's Love

We become defeated in any effort when despair leads us to conclude that some areas of life lie outside the circle of God's love. This kind of thinking compartmentalizes God and limits expectation of His care.

What a mistake!

God's love extends to every part of life and even employs each experience we face to prove His goodness to us: "And we know that all things work together for good to them that love God, to them who are the called according to His purpose" (Rom. 8:28).

When it became clear to me that God wanted to meet overweight people in their need, I began a study of Bible texts that seemed to offer hope to those longing to lose weight. Soon I had enough evidence to present my case to a class, and from that small beginning grew a book entitled *Weight! A Better Way to Lose* and a cassette series that have made their way around the world, helping many achieve their goals in weight control.

An atheist in France surprised his overweight wife by saying, "If your God can enable you to lose eighty pounds, I will go to church with you."

Her pastor wrote for my book and cassettes on weight control, and his last letter assured me that the atheist will soon have to start attending church with his wife or eat his words.

But was this doubting husband's challenge a valid expectation of his wife's Christianity?

Absolutely.

Why shouldn't the world expect our faith to work wherever it is needed?

If you have been taking your weight lightly, it is time to get serious about your problem and realize that God cares about this very personal part of your life.

Test this truth by thinking about your feelings toward those you love.

Do you care when they hurt?

Of course you do . . . even if you might sometimes prefer to shut their problems out of your mind. When you love people, you care about their difficulties. Indifference and love are incompatible.

And God loves us: "Herein is love, not that we loved God, but that He loved us, and sent His Son to be the propitiation for our sins" (1 John 4:10).

The death of Christ on the cross ought to settle any insecurity we might have about God's love: "But God commendeth

His love toward us, in that while we were yet sinners, Christ died for us" (Rom. 5:8).

We may be sure then that our Lord cares about all of our hurts and understands them. If you are distressed about being overweight, you can be certain that God wants to meet you in this very sensitive area of your life and there demonstrate His love.

A Christian weight control class member wrote to me saying the group had lost a total of 1,000 pounds, using my book and tapes as study guides. Later, another card came saying the group had lost 2,000 pounds. Finally, a third message arrived boosting the total class losses to 4,000 pounds. Needless to say, I was pleased to accept an invitation to speak at one of the meetings of this thriving class.

When I entered the church basement room where the class held its meetings, I found it decorated with tokens of their successes. Photographs of members were posted, which showed them before and after their discovery that a biblical lifestyle could make a difference in conquering weight problems.

Clothing displays on the walls demonstrated the changes in size of successful class members. The general atmosphere of the class was positive and enthusiastic. But most moving to me was the personal story of a woman whose search for a way to lose weight had ended in one disappointment after another until she learned that God cares about all of her needs and desires, even her longing to be thin and trim. She had found her new look in the Old Book and this changed her life. If you are troubled about being overweight, that same discovery can make it possible for you to lose those unwanted pounds and become the person you want to be.

God's Love Is Shown in His Creation

I begin each day by quoting the following Bible verses:

> Behold the fowls of the air: for they sow not, neither
> do they reap, nor gather into barns; yet your Heavenly

Father feedeth them. Are ye not much better than they? (Matt. 6:26)

And why take ye thought for raiment? Consider the lilies of the field, how they grow; they toil not, neither do they spin: And yet I say unto you, that even Solomon in all his glory was not arrayed like one of these. Wherefore, if God so clothe the grass of the field, which today is, and tomorrow is cast into the oven, shall He not much more clothe you, O ye of little faith? (Matt. 6:28-30)

But seek ye first the kingdom of God, and His righteousness; and all these things shall be added unto you (Matt. 6:33).

Quoting these faith-building verses reminds me that God's love is revealed in all of His creation and that nothing in my life escapes His view. The smallest problem I face is important to Him.

If God cares about the appearance of lilies that are seen for a few weeks and then wither and die, my appearance must be important to Him.

If I mean more to my Heavenly Father than fowl or flowers, He must care about my success in achieving sensible weight control, an issue that can affect me both physically and emotionally, possibly either shortening or lengthening my life.

The Metropolitan Life Insurance Company issued this stern warning to those who have thought being overweight doesn't really matter: *"For every inch your waist measurement exceeds your chest measurement, subtract two years from your life."*

SUBTRACT TWO YEARS FROM YOUR LIFE!

That's a loss you can do without.

A missionary who was overweight received a letter, from one of her superiors in the mission, that quickly changed her lifestyle and appearance. The letter simply expressed regret that the maxi-missionary would have such a brief time to serve her Lord on the mission field since her life would be shortened by her excess weight.

The dangers of obesity are well-known and will be emphasized later. For now, just remember that being overweight makes you a more likely candidate for heart disease, high blood pressure, diabetes, strokes, gallbladder problems, complications during childbirth, and even cancer.

Our Bodies Created as His Temple

God's love for us is revealed in the special care He took in creating our bodies. Everything in the universe, except the human body, was simply spoken into existence: "And God said, 'Let the earth bring forth the living creature after his kind, cattle, and creeping thing, and beast of the earth after its kind': and it was so" (Gen. 1:24).

Not so the body of man. Here our Lord's creative method was modified to show His love and care:

> And God said, "Let us make man in our image, after our likeness: and let them have dominion over the fish of the sea, and over the fowl of the air, and over the cattle, and over all the earth, and over every creeping thing that creepeth upon the earth" (Gen. 1:26).
>
> And the Lord God formed man of the dust of the ground, and breathed into his nostrils the breath of life; and man became a living soul (Gen. 2:7).

The Psalmist David also acknowledged the miracle of creation revealed in our bodies and wrote: "I will praise Thee; for I am fearfully and wonderfully made" (Ps. 139:14).

When Christ came to earth to bring us salvation, He chose the human body as His vehicle of redemption. He was "made in the likeness of men" (Phil. 2:7). He referred to His body as His *temple* and said the resurrection of His body would be the proof of His deity (John 2:18-22).

Christ was resurrected bodily from the grave, just as we shall be at His return. This coming resurrection reveals divine regard for our bodies.

> But now is Christ risen from the dead, and become the
> firstfruits of them that slept. For since by man came
> death, by man came also the resurrection of the dead.
> For as in Adam all die, even so in Christ shall all be
> made alive. But every man in his own order: Christ the
> firstfruits; afterward they that are Christ's at His com-
> ing (1 Cor. 15:20-23).

When that day arrives, our bodies will be perfect without
the need of diets or doctors.

Till then, calories count.

Most encouraging to the Christian should be the fact that
his/her body is the temple of God. The Bible teaches that the
Holy Spirit actually lives within every believer. Jesus promised:

> And I will pray the Father, and He shall give you an-
> other Comforter, that He may abide with you for ever;
> even the Spirit of Truth; whom the world cannot re-
> ceive, because it seeth Him not, neither knoweth Him:
> but ye know Him; for He dwelleth with you, and shall
> be in you (John 14:16-17).

Paul confirmed the fulfilling of our Lord's promise by writing: "What? Know ye not that your body is the temple of the
Holy Ghost which is in you, which ye have of God, and ye are
not your own? For ye are bought with a price: therefore,
glorify God in your body and in your spirit, which are God's"
(1 Cor. 6:19-20).

Think of it! Your body is the house of God.

A group of teens broke into a church building in a Michigan
city and vandalized it. They poured paint over the organ and
pulpit and generally desecrated this house of worship.

The community was outraged, demanding justice.

But many Christians regularly mistreat their bodies, forget-
ting that each one is God's sanctuary.

Pastor Knute Larson of "The Chapel" in Akron, Ohio
brought this important teaching home to his congregation

through the following pastoral note in the church bulletin:

> Thank you for bringing the sanctuary ... into the
> church building today. If you are a Christian, that is
> exactly what has happened.
>   We have brought our sanctuaries, God's dwelling
> places, into the building set aside for the church to
> meet.

So now you have a divine dimension to a disciplined lifestyle. Since your body is the Lord's temple, it should be kept in
the best possible condition at all times.

Some Christians miss this truth. They seem to think it carnal
to be concerned about personal appearance. Weight control is
something relegated to "the flesh." They leave the impression
that their goals are higher.

These same people will work long and give sacrificially to
make the local church building attractive. After all, it is the
Lord's house. Yet, nowhere in the New Testament is this title
given to a meeting place for the church. Instead, your *body* is
called the temple of God.

The principal reason for not conquering your weight problem may be a mistaken separation of the physical and spiritual.
To you, spiritual dedication has to do with singing in the
choir, going to church services, praying, reading your Bible,
and witnessing to your neighbors about their need of receiving Christ as Saviour.

While these acts of service and worship are certainly important ingredients of the Christian life, they do not rule out
taking proper care of your body. If your health fails, your
opportunity for sacred service will be severely limited.

Besides, to the Christian, everything is to be sacred:

> Therefore if any man be in Christ, he is a new crea-
> ture: old things are passed away; behold all things are
> become new. And all things are of God, who hath

reconciled us to Himself by Jesus Christ, and hath given to us the ministry of reconciliation (2 Cor. 5:17-18).

Commitment to Christ calls for a complete surrender of all—including our bodies: "I beseech you therefore, brethren, by the mercies of God, that ye present your bodies a living sacrifice, holy, acceptable unto God, which is your reasonable service" (Rom. 12:1).

Since your body is the temple of the Holy Spirit, it is logical to conclude that His power is available for the purpose of keeping it in a condition that is pleasing to Him. It is His property.

You can claim God's power in your effort to take proper care of His temple. Recognizing this, a number of Christian weight control classes have included the word *temple* in their class name.

Many who have started giving attention to keeping their temples trim have been surprised to find that a new appreciation for God's temple has brought many other positive changes in their lives. This is what happened to Judy Kurnik.

Judy Kurnik's Surprise

Judy had attended Bible college, intending to enter Christian service, but her future did not unfold as she had planned. Frustrated and depressed, she finally sought help from her pastor. He saw her overweight condition as a key to her problems and gave her my book, *Weight! A Better Way to Lose.* When good things began to happen in Judy's life as a result of facing up to her need of a new lifestyle that would enable her to achieve weight control, she sent me the following letter:

*I cannot begin to thank you enough for the book **Weight! A Better Way to Lose.** The impact that it has had upon my life has been tremendous! I was in counseling with my pastor (in a seemingly futile attempt to establish a Christian life after 18 years of running from God) when the Lord laid* *it on his heart to give me your book. The poor man must have done so with much fear since my temper and depression were my greatest problems!*

I took the book home, totally humiliated that anyone would think that weight was the basis of my spiritual problems. After reading a few pages I realized that the weight was my way of punishing myself for having turned my back on full-time Christian service.

The Lord spoke to me on every page of that book! Many "talks" followed with the pastor and with each God revealed new areas of my life to deal with. Each area was covered in your book, and over the months it has been a constant source of help to me. I have gone from being a totally depressed person with a terrible marriage to a happy, submissive Christian woman who adores her husband and children and finds it increasingly difficult to remember what the "old person" was even like.

Jesus has become more than my Saviour—He is my sweet and precious Lord! He loved me when I couldn't love myself.

At this point, I have lost 92 pounds with 98 more to go. I have the Christian home and family that was always my dream, and the Lord has led me into areas of ministry where the agony of my past is helping others.

I have a long way to go in repairing the extreme physical damage I caused myself (Pastor refers to it as my "rebuilding the temple!"), but each day in that way is precious to me. Gone are the hatred and bitterness, and love has taken their place.

I guess in all this, my greatest moment of joy came when I looked into the mirror one morning and realized that I had totally forgiven myself for my past and that I really liked— no, that I really loved the person that God has allowed me to become!

> *Sincerely in Jesus,*
> *Judy Kurnik*

[handwritten notes: Reject — Oh Well I goofed up I might as well forget about it. Satan / I can't do this! / wrong Jesus name]

Our Compassionate Lord

A woman who attended one of my Spiritual Life and Weight Control seminars said she felt that I had a genuine concern for those who were trying to lose weight and that this had been of help to her. I hope she was correct for there would be no way to project the compassion of Christ for those in need without feeling it.

To be compassionate is to feel the pain and distress of another.

Have you noticed the many Bible references to the Lord's unfailing compassion?

Consider some of them.

The Prophet Jeremiah revealed that the Lord's compassions are proof of His faithfulness and that they are new every morning: "It is of the Lord's mercies that we are not consumed, because His compassions fail not. They are new every morning: great is thy faithfulness" (Lam. 3:22-23).

Jesus was often moved with compassion because of the needs of the multitudes He met along the way: "But when He saw the multitudes, He was moved with compassion on them, because they fainted, and were scattered abroad, as sheep having no shepherd" (Matt. 9:36).

Lepers were cleansed (Matt. 8:2-4).

The blind received their sight (Matt. 9:27-31).

Little children were blessed (Matt. 19:13-15).

The lame were made to walk (Matt. 11:5).

The dead were raised to life again (Luke 7:11-15).

Our compassionate Lord wept at the grave of Lazarus (John 11:35) and mourned over the sorrows that would come to the people of Jerusalem because of their rejection of His offer of salvation (Luke 19:41-44).

And here you are wondering if He cares about a problem that eats away at you continually, a problem that robs you of peace of mind and the power to achieve your full potential in life.

Of course He cares!

The Bible guarantees it.

But there is another who must care if you are to achieve your goal of consistent weight control.

You must care!

It's Your Move

You are the foot soldier in this weight war. Without your full participation, the battle will be lost. Help is available, but you must reach for it.

So the ball has just been passed to you.

What are you going to do about it?

Do you really want to lose weight?

Is your appearance important to you?

Do you believe that your weight may be adversely affecting your health?

Is weight robbing you of the joy of living?

Do you envy people who always seem to look just right?

Are you spending money to take off pounds? Have you ever done so in the past?

Could weight be affecting your Christian testimony?

Have you been neglecting God's temple?

Now for the most important question of all: Are you willing to change the way you live? If not, the biblical instruction on weight control that I am about to share with you will be little more than a reading exercise.

Five years from today you will probably be starting another grapefruit diet, or some other fruity fad. You will have bounced your way through a score of yo-yo experiences on the bathroom scales without getting one ounce closer to the answer you have been seeking. And you will still be looking for some effortless way to become thin and trim.

On the other hand, you may finally be tired of the gimmicks and false promises of the quick-fix diets. You want the real thing, even if it involves a revolution in your way of life. If so, you may be ready to embark on a great adventure in self-control and positive living that will enable you to shed those unwanted pounds and taste the joy of living every day on higher ground.

Questions for Application

1. What are the benefits of having a "trim temple"?

2. How is the approach to dieting suggested in this chapter different than other methods you have tried?

God's help - comforter - God's on my side all I can be

3. What characteristics of God assure you that He cares about your struggle to lose weight?

- Compassionate -
- He made us
- love us
- cares for us

(Triggers) & how to stop them.

① Bring picture of when you liked how you looked — what size were you then?

② What is your goal

③ What life style changes will you work out to accomplish your goal?

2

Is It Wrong to Long to Be Thin?

Speak to some people of dieting or trying to lose weight, and you will get an immediate negative response. They react this way for a number of reasons.

A husband of an overweight woman may fear losing his wife to another man if she becomes slim and trim.

Some parents rest easier if their daughters are overweight just enough to thin down the number of young men who are interested in them.

Others see efforts to lose weight as carnal and unimportant since spiritual matters should have priority over physical matters.

What is the proper attitude toward weight control?

Is it ever wrong to long to be thin?

It is certainly possible to have wrong motives for desiring to lose weight.

The Pharisees gave gifts to the poor so that others would be impressed by their supposed generosity. Although these gifts were undoubtedly needed and appreciated by those who received them, Jesus rebuked the Pharisees for their constant grandstanding and called them hypocrites (Matt. 6:2).

Good works that spring from bad motives are sinful. And motives are expressions of the heart.

Both Jesus and James gave examples of even prayer becoming sinful when the motives for praying are wrong.

> And when thou prayest, thou shalt not be as the hypocrites are: for they love to pray standing in the synagogues and in the corners of the streets, that they may be seen of men. Verily I say unto you, they have their reward (Matt. 6:5).

> Ye ask, and receive not, because ye ask amiss, that ye may consume it upon your lusts (James 4:3).

If prayer can become sinful when improperly motivated, this must also be true of trying to lose weight. Under some conditions it is wrong to long to be thin.

Wrong Motives for Losing Weight

It is wrong to desire to lose weight to provoke lust. In the New Testament the word *lust* is usually a translation of the Greek word *epthumia,* meaning "a passionate craving." When this passionate craving calls for breaking the moral law of God, it becomes evil desire.

Solomon tells of an immoral woman who invites a young man into her home to commit adultery (Prov. 7:7-23). She has her mind set on seducing this man and prepares for it.

She dresses to seduce.

She goes into the street at night where she knows he will pass and offers herself to him, assuring him that her husband is away on a business trip and that he will not return that night.

She even describes the preparation of her bed for his visit.

> I have decked my bed with coverings of tapestry, with carved works, with fine linen of Egypt. I have perfumed my bed with myrrh, aloes, and cinnamon.

Come, let us take our fill of love until the morning: let us solace ourselves with loves. For the goodman is not at home, he is gone a long journey: He hath taken a bag of money with him, and will come home at the day appointed (Prov. 7:16-20).

There is, of course, nothing wrong with making a bed beautiful; nothing sinful about coverings of tapestry and fine linen.

Perfume the sheets if you please ... and if it pleases your spouse.

But when the motivation for all of these preparations is immoral, you have made a bad bed.

Provoking lust is always wrong, even when it masquerades as a desire for attractiveness and health. If lust is your motivation for losing weight, it will be wrong for you to long to be thin.

Longing to lose weight will also be wrong for you if your motivation for losing is personal pride.

Now our study is becoming sensitive.

Pride is popular today, even among Christians. Many overweight people have felt inferior for so long that pride over becoming thin may seem justified.

Have you been longing for a time when you can outshine your thin friends whom you have been resenting, and who always seem to look just right?

Have you been waiting to get even?

Have you been fantasizing about showing off your new trim look in their presence and for once getting all the attention?

Your feelings, though understandable, have their roots in pride. Self-exaltation is always harmful and is best conquered by cultivating an attitude of gratitude for all achievements.

See how serious pride is to God:

The fear of the Lord is to hate evil: pride, and arrogancy, and the evil way, and the froward mouth, do I hate (Prov. 8:13).

When pride cometh, then cometh shame: but with

the lowly is wisdom (Prov. 11:2).

Love not the world, neither the things that are in the world. If any man love the world, the love of the Father is not in him. For all that is in the world, the lust of the flesh, and the lust of the eyes, and the pride of life, is not of the Father, but is of the world (1 John 2:15-16).

Could it be that you have failed to get your weight under control because your motive to lose has been pride? Has a lack of humility kept you from needed self-control that comes from a selfless yielding to the Holy Spirit? Measuring the pride factor in your life might be the key to success in losing those unwanted pounds.

Finally, it is wrong to long to be thin when losing weight may jeopardize your health.

While losing weight is usually healthful, an obsession with slimness can cost the diligent dieter his or her health; sometimes the drive to be thin has even led to death. This is especially true among those who have become the victims of anorexia nervosa, an eating disorder that usually afflicts young women in their middle or upper teenage years.

In her article, "Anorexia Nervosa: I Almost Starved to Death," Dianne Lawson tells of being so addicted to dieting that she counted every calorie she consumed, including those in the toothpaste she was using. Sometimes she would go two or three days without food to make up for eating a meal she could not avoid.

Dianne had started dieting to lose a few pounds, wanting to get down to 108. But before her ordeal was over she weighed only 70 pounds and had to be hospitalized to save her life.

At the time she entered the hospital, Dianne was having severe circulation problems and was fainting frequently. She says her skin had become ashen gray, and her blood pressure was very low. Her fingernails had seemingly ceased to grow. Her body had begun consuming her own muscles for nutrients and in the process had damaged her heart.

Thankfully, Dianne has recovered and as a result of her experience says she has come into a new relationship with her family and with God. While she once thought of God as a supreme taskmaster, she now knows Him as the One who loves her and understands when she is alone or in need. Others have not been so fortunate and have permanently damaged their health by anorexic behavior. Some have died.[1]

While most victims of eating disorders are from middle-class and upper-class homes, recent research indicates that eating problems are showing up in all economic classes and age-groups.

Studies indicate that 95 percent of eating disorder victims are women. As many as one out of five women in college may be either anorexic or bulimic (a condition where the victim is obsessed with both food and weight, leading to bouts of gorging and self-induced vomiting).[2] Up to 20 percent of women between the ages of fifteen and thirty are victims.[3] Males, however, are also becoming subject to eating disorders with increasing frequency.

In their book, *There's More to Being Thin Than Being Thin,* Neva Coyle and Marie Chapian explain:

> The anorexic or bulimic person has exaggerated fears of becoming fat, even though she is close to normal weight. A high percentage of people with these eating disorders are women. They overreact to society's dictates of beauty and femininity and feel exaggerated pressures to be thin.[4]

In her article, "Dying to Be Thin," published in *Family Circle* magazine, Caroline Adams Miller describes her seven-year nightmare as a victim of bulimia and says she had come to blame society for expecting women not only to be bright, witty, exuberant, and beautiful, but also to fit into size-4 designer jeans.[5]

This common thread of trying to live up to the expectations of others seems to run through most of the stories of those who long to be thin to the point of jeopardizing their health and risking their lives to achieve it. They feel they must conform to the pressure of their peers, their families, or society even if it destroys them.

Do not embark on any weight loss program for the wrong reasons, including a desire to please others or to conform to the image of the so-called beautiful people who flaunt their figures and builds on television screens and the covers of magazines. God loves you as you are, and if you truly need to lose weight, He will enable you to do so in a way that will contribute to the good health and the abundant life He desires for you.*

Now that we've considered some of the wrong reasons for wanting to lose weight, let's look at the positive side of sensible weight control. Generally it is not wrong to long to be thin.

Knowing How Thin You Should Be

Longing to lose weight is not wrong when you weigh more than you should for your height and frame.

Size and weight charts are available from your doctor and at many bookstores. According to the Mayo Clinic, however, you may not have to diet despite what the height-weight charts say if you have a sense of energy and well-being, normal blood pressure, normal triglyceride and cholesterol levels, and if you are satisfied with the way you look.

Consulting with your family doctor about what you should weigh, considering your height and frame, will be time and money well spent.

After you have gathered all this information, remember that you are unique and that you are important to God. You have a special place in His plan, and finding that place is more important than conforming to the dimensions of a skinny world.

---

*In the back of this book, I have listed several organizations that offer information about eating disorders. If you have symptoms of an eating disorder, or know that someone you love has them, contact a doctor immediately.

I visited a man a number of times in an effort to lead him to faith in Christ. He had been quite successful as a farmer and businessman but now was rather withdrawn from social contacts. He always seemed to appreciate my visits and concern for him, yet he would not respond to my message.

Finally, I discovered the reason for his reluctance: he was afraid that in coming to faith in Christ he would lose his individuality. He feared that salvation would make him "just another Christian, one of the crowd headed for heaven."

Nothing could be farther from the truth.

It is true that God loves the world, but He loves you as an individual. There is a particular place for you in the body of Christ that no one else can fill. Your gifts and talents have been given to you so that you can carry out your role in the church.

> For the body is not one member, but many. If the foot shall say, because I am not the hand, I am not of the body; is it therefore not of the body? And if the ear shall say, because I am not the eye, I am not of the body; is it therefore not of the body? If the whole body were an eye, where were the hearing? If the whole were hearing, where were the smelling? But now hath God set the members every one of them in the body, as it hath pleased Him (1 Cor. 12:14-18).

Each of us is equipped exactly as God intends for our good and His glory, including the height and frame He has given us which should always be kept at its best.

When my friend saw that he was unique in God's eyes, he was ready to receive Christ as his Lord and Saviour. He wanted to get in on God's plan for his life.

Your uniqueness is precious to your Heavenly Father.

Accepting this truth will set you free.

The Dangers of Obesity
Desiring to lose weight in order to improve your health and

lengthen your life will always be right.

Being overweight can be deadly.

Dr. Jules Hirsch, chairman of a fourteen member panel of doctors and nutritionists assembled by the National Institute of Health, called obesity a killer that is just as dangerous to health as smoking. As reported in *Time* magazine, Dr. Hirsch warned that the public tends to regard obestiy as something more involved with appearance than health but that in reality it is a very pervasive health hazard in many systems of the body.

Explaining some conclusions of the panel, Claudia Wallis writes:

> According to the panel, the hazards become significant for a person who is 20 percent or more above the desirable weight as determined by the Metropolitan Life Insurance tables. By these standards, about 34 million American adults and one out of every five people over age nineteen are obese. Of these, 11 million qualify as severely obese because they exceed their desirable weights by 40 percent or more.

What are the specific dangers to these overweight people?

They have three times the normal incidence of high blood pressure and diabetes, an increased risk of heart disease, a shorter lifespan, and an unusually high risk of developing respiratory disorders, arthritis, and certain types of cancer.

A severely obese woman, for example, has five times the normal risk of developing cancer of the uterine lining and an increased risk of breast and cervical cancers. Men who are significantly overweight have an increased chance of developing malignancies of the colon, rectum, and prostate.

Hirsch, a professor at Rockefeller University, added another shocker by saying that relatively small amounts of excess flab, even five pounds, can be dangerous, particularly to people already at risk for hypertension and diabetes.

And here's a surprise: where you carry your extra weight

can influence your health. Studies show that people who pack their flab as a potbelly or a spare tire are more apt to suffer from heart disease, stroke, and diabetes than those who carry the same amount around their hips and thighs. This may chalk up another point for the value of exercise.

All of these warnings by the experts have led *Time* reporter, Claudia Wallis, to wonder if in the future we may see the following warning on candy wrappers and refrigerator doors: THE SURGEON GENERAL HAS DETERMINED THAT OBESITY IS DANGEROUS TO YOUR HEALTH.[6]

The Good Life

Slimming down then, may contribute more to life than a good feeling when looking in the mirror. According to respected health authorities, taking off extra pounds contributes to good health and probably to the length of life.

Richard Ely, a busy pastor, has been tasting the joy of improved health and increased vigor since he recognized being overweight was a spiritual problem and set out to conquer it. In a letter to me describing his new way of life, he says:

I had been struggling with my health for five or six years. It was beginning to take a toll on my ability to keep up with my responsibilities in the ministry and at home. The more stress I experienced, the more I ate, and the problem just kept growing. I found myself worn out by two or three in the afternoon with many more hours still to go.

I had to admit that it was a spiritual problem for me, food was an escape for me from the stress and pressure of the ministry.

Pastor Ely cut down his calorie intake and gained strength to do so daily by committing his problem to the Lord. He found the first three days to be the most crucial because of experiencing withdrawal from sugar and feelings of hunger, but he persevered and has been successful in losing his excess weight. But reducing calories was only part of his program.

Exercise was equally important. He wrote:

I began a walking program, one to two miles a day and gradually worked up to thirty to forty miles per week after three months, and I did fifty to seventy-five sit-ups per day.

I've lost fifty pounds and feel like a new person at home and at work. I've been involved in physical activities that I gave up ten years ago, and I'm enjoying them also. I feel better about myself, and I now realize that Satan was defeating me in this area of my life, and I didn't realize it.

I have people tell me they can't afford the time, but this isn't valid. They can't afford not to spend the time.

The key is maintenance. I've told myself most people can go on a diet and lose it, but keeping it off is the key. I'm maintaining my desired weight by keeping up my walking, and I'm eating about 2,500 calories a day. I've discovered that the time walking is a precious time when I can talk and listen to the Lord and enjoy the beauty of His creation.

You must structure your diet and exercise program to fit you. That is critical if you are going to be successful. Also, realize you have a serious problem and treat it as a spiritual struggle.

> *In Christ,*
> *Richard Ely*

When your goal in losing weight is better health, you have proper motivation, and it is not wrong to long to be thin. But there is another proper reason for longing to lose: the desire to demonstrate the power of God working in and through you, enhancing your personal witness for Christ and bringing glory to God.

To God Be the Glory

Bill Pauley, a minister, weighed 384 pounds and had a 58-inch waist. He said that buying a car was like buying a suit—he had to be fitted. When he wanted to weigh himself, he went to the butcher shop to use the scale. He recalled:

> I will always remember the time I boarded the air-
> plane and sat in one of those tight seats. I could hardly
> get into it. When the stewardess asked if my seatbelt
> was fastened, I told her I could not get it around me in
> the first place; and in the second place, if there were a
> crash, she would not have to worry—I would be stuck
> to the seat permanently!

For the most part, Bill had been able to laugh off his heavy-
weight appearance. He seems to have followed the if-you-
have-a-lemon-make-lemonade policy, and he had even developed a fine string of jokes about his weight to use as openers
in his meetings. Then one day he found himself in a situation
that wasn't funny.

While he was the speaker in youth meetings in central Illi-
nois, he heard about a statement made by one of the teenage
girls there. She had said, "If Mr. Pauley can eat, then I can
smoke."

That girl's observation was an eye-opener to Pauley. Later
he said, "For years I had criticized smoking and drinking and
had preached the Word of God without applying the matter of
temperance to myself. It was not until I heard what this girl
had said that I became convicted of overeating."

Bill Pauley claimed the power of God and went on a diet.
He lost 179 pounds, and his waist went from 58 inches to 36
inches. He ended his weight problem and gained the victory
as a demonstration of the power of God working in him. His
success in this formerly neglected area of his life improved his
witness for Christ and brought glory to God.[7]

In one church where I ministered, the Sunday School superintendent and the church pianist were husband and wife and
were both overweight. A class was started in the church using
my book *Weight! A Better Way to Lose* and my weight control seminar on cassettes. Both the superintendent and the
pianist joined the class and began losing weight.

Each Sunday the superintendent and the pianist came before the congregation to carry out their service for the Lord and were thinner than the week before. The whole church began to rejoice in what God was doing in their lives, and on the Sunday they announced a total weight loss between them of 100 pounds, the congregation broke into applause over their victory. Their newfound discipline was a good testimony to their church of deeper commitment to Christ. And God was glorified.

There are many gains in achieving desired weight control: improved health, fewer emotional hang-ups, even a longer life, to name a few. But the most important reason for losing weight may be the impact your new lifestyle has on others as you demonstrate God's power working in you, making it possible for you to become the disciplined person you need to be to conquer your weight problem. When that is your goal, you can be sure it is not wrong to long to be thin.

Questions for Application

1. Pastor Ely said that being overweight was a spiritual problem for him. How do you react to this statement?

2. If a friend or family member has anorexia, what symptoms would you notice? What symptoms could help you identify a bulimic person?

3. Can you think of other wrong motives for losing weight that were not discussed in this chapter?

4. How can success in weight control affect your relationship to God?

3

Which Diet Works?

Sharp jabbing pains knifed into the left side of my chest, making it difficult to breathe. At first, I was not too concerned because I had suffered from these attacks periodically throughout most of my life, especially during times of stress or heavy exertion. And today had been particularly taxing.

In addition to caring for my usual duties as the pastor of a large suburban church, I had made a trip to Metropolitan Airport, about forty miles from my home, so that a friend could catch a plane to New York. After helping with heavy baggage, I had fought my way back through bustling Detroit rush hour traffic to get home for other responsibilities.

My discomfort had started about 11 P.M., just as we were finishing up the day. The pattern was familiar: pulsating pains in my chest, prohibiting deep breathing. On other occasions, these had subsided within five to fifteen minutes, bringing great relief. But tonight was different. The pains persisted and after a time were accompanied by nausea, so I decided to go to the hospital.

Upon arriving at the emergency room of the hospital, I was

given a number of tests: X rays, electrocardiogram, etc. Finally, the examining physician explained that there was nothing wrong with my heart and that the pain had been caused by muscle spasms. He suspected that I had been working too hard and assured me that a shot of a muscle relaxant would take care of everything.

The shot certainly was relaxing. I slept most of the time for the next few days, had no more pain, and soon felt quite well again.

But I was not well.

The cause of my problem had not been treated, only the symptoms. And as the months passed, other symptoms began to appear. Many of these were emotional and this disturbed me. Staying calm became a battle. Little problems seemed insurmountable. Irritations that I would normally have cared for with ease and then forgotten bothered me for days. At times, tears burned in my eyes, and the lump in my throat wouldn't go away.

Though I had considered myself a positive person, a cloud of depression now began to hover over me. I found myself speaking sharply to members of my family. Fears became my constant companions. Driving in heavy traffic began to bother me, and crowded buildings brought a feeling of panic. Often I would awaken in the night, sweating and trembling. Twice I endorsed checks during those traumatic times so that my family would have money in the event of my death before morning.

Fortunately, three or four months after my emergency room visit, my doctor correctly diagnosed my condition as hypoglycemia (low blood sugar) and advised a change in my eating habits. Hypoglycemia is triggered by sugar intake which causes the body to produce too much insulin.

Now I would begin a new chapter in my life: I would learn to live on a special diet. Some scoff at the thought of ever living on a diet. Yet everyone does. A diet simply sets the limits on the type and quantity of food you can eat. These limits may be broad or confined for a special purpose.

Special Diets in the Bible

Our first parents received a special diet from their Creator. This diet provided for great variety in eating and had but one restriction: they could eat the fruit of every tree in the Garden of Eden except the fruit of the tree of the knowledge of good and evil (Gen. 2:16-17).

Obedience, not obesity, was the issue when Adam and Eve disobeyed the Lord and ate the forbidden fruit, but food was certaintly a factor in that first temptation, and we should not forget it.

For their journey from Egypt to Canaan, the Children of Israel were given a diet of manna and meat. Both were miraculously supplied (Ex. 16:13-15). As far as we know this was the only time that men have shared the diet of angels (Ps. 78:25).

Dietary laws were an important part of the instructions given to Moses for his people to observe in their new land. With regard to meats, they were allowed to eat any animal that parted the hoof and chewed the cud. Other animals were to be considered unclean. Great detail was also given to describing how to recognize the clean and unclean of fish and fowl (Deut. 14:3-21). These laws of diet were to set the nation of Israel apart from other nations.

Christians are not bound by dietary laws today. Paul declared our freedom from them as the result of the death of Christ on the cross (Col. 2:16-17). Nevertheless, the dietary laws recorded in the Old Testament demonstrate the biblical principle of special diets for certain worthwhile purposes.

More examples are worth noting.

As a Nazarite, Samson drank neither wine nor strong drink and abstained from eating any unclean thing (Jud. 13:4).

Daniel and his friends chose vegetarian fare instead of the meat that had been offered them by Nebuchadnezzar. At the end of ten days, they were healthier than those who ate from the king's menu (Dan. 1:15).

John the Baptist lived on locusts and wild honey. That was an unusual diet, but John was an unusual man.

Learning to Live without Sugar

Like the first diet given to man, mine had but one restriction. In my case, that restriction was sugar. And I was to learn that eliminating sugar from my diet was no easy task.

To help you understand my difficulty, let me tell you about my eating habits before becoming sugar free:

My practice had been to start each morning with coffee, cereal, and toast. The coffee and cereal were sweetened to my taste with sugar or honey, and the toast was liberally spread with jelly. In midmorning, I had coffee and a glazed donut or two. Lunch was capped with cookies or cake when possible, and when these were not available, I ate another slice of bread and jelly. My sweet tooth demanded attention at some time during the afternoon, not only because of my craving for the taste of something sweet, but because my energy level would be very low at that time of day. Often dinner was rounded out with a piece of pie, and before going to bed I usually ate a dish of ice cream or some other sweet snack.

"Cut back on sugar," my doctor said. When I did this, there was some improvement, and I was given a glucose tolerance test which confirmed the hypoglycemia. This meant ending my sugar spree for the rest of my life.

Gone were sugar and honey to sweeten my breakfast.

Gone were glazed donuts in midmorning.

No more cookies or cupcakes for lunch.

No more candy bars in the afternoon.

Desserts would be absent from dinner.

Evening snack times would never be sweet again.

Was this drastic diet change difficult for me to achieve?

Yes. It became one of the toughest challenges of my life. I still remember watching my hand tremble when I wanted to reach for a glass of soda pop that I knew contained sugar and therefore was off-limits for me.

"Now you know what I was going through when I was trying to stop smoking," a friend said.

I had often sympathized with people in bondage to habits and had sometimes quoted Paul's declaration of independence to them: "I will not be brought under the power of any" (1 Cor. 6:12). But now I was learning firsthand about the power of an addiction to food, a bondage I had never imagined having before beginning that personal struggle to be free.

Did I win the battle over sugar addiction?

Absolutely.

God has equipped every believer to win. I simply had to deepen my devotional life and claim the power of God to be victorious over temptation. Since Jesus Himself entered the arena of temptation and emerged victorious, He is able to understand the struggles encountered by those who belong to Him and enable them to overcome (Heb. 4:15-16).

Upon changing my way of eating, the frightening symptoms I had been experiencing began to decline and finally ceased. Along with this improvement in health came an added bonus that I had not anticipated: I began to lose weight.

Though I did not have a serious weight problem (my wife said you could only tell by hugging), I had begun to gain easily, and my waist had increased by four sizes. After age forty, I had added twenty-five pounds, and had I not changed my lifestyle, I believe the future would have found me a well-rounded person.

In addition, the weight that I had gained seemed to settle mostly around my waist. I recall standing before a mirror one day and feeling as if my chest had been moving down on me.

"Something really does happen after forty," I had said.

Eliminating sugar from my diet changed all that. I lost all I had gained, and though I am now sixty-seven, I have regained the approximate weight and build that I had before I started gaining weight in my forties.

While I abstain from high carbohydrate foods such as pie, cake, cookies, and other such goodies, there are many acceptable and delicious foods available to me, and I concentrate on these rather than on my one restriction.

I can eat steaks, chops, seafoods, poultry, vegetables, dairy products, and most unsweetened fruits. This diet allows a fine variety of healthful and enjoyable food, and the satisfaction that comes from practicing self-control is dessert enough for me.

The following is a sample of my diet on an average day.

Breakfast	eggs or egg substitute (no cholesterol) Toast—one slice with old-fashioned peanut butter Decaffeinated coffee without sugar Unsweetened fruit
Midmorning	Low fat milk
Lunch	Soup Meat sandwich Salad Cottage cheese Decaffeinated coffee without sugar
Midafternoon	Low fat milk and peanuts
Dinner	Meat Vegetable Salad Cottage cheese Unsweetened fruit One slice of bread with margarine Decaffeinated coffee without sugar
Evening snack	Low fat milk or cold cuts

With minor variations, I have stayed with the above way of eating for many, many years and have no desire to change. I have found a lifestyle with which I am comfortable and am content to continue it for the rest of my life.

The Mayo Clinic Approach

I believe the "rest of my life" test is a good one for any diet, and I am not alone in this view. Experts at the Mayo Clinic feel that "dieting" implies something you do only until you succeed or fail. The danger of this kind of thinking is that either way you're going to return to your former eating patterns which caused you to gain weight in the first place. They prefer a permanent way of eating that provides proper nourishment and keeps weight in a desired range.

The Mayo Clinic approach is to tailor menus to individuals, but the general plan divides food into six groups: protein (meat, fish, poultry, cheese), milk, starches, vegetables, fruits, and fats and oils. Fifty-five percent of our daily caloric intake should be derived from carbohydrates. Most of these calories should come from complex carbohydrates found in a variety of foods, such as, potatoes, breads, pastas, rice, and other whole grains as opposed to simple carbohydrates that are in sugary foods like cookies, cakes, and candies.

While crash diets often go as low as 800 calories a day, the Mayo Clinic plan provides approximately 1,400 calories daily, depending on the needs and activity of the person desiring to lose weight.[1]

Diets, Diets, Diets, Diets

While there are many weight loss diets offered today, they seem to fall into four categories: fad diets, low-sugar diets, low-fat diets, and calorie-counting diets.

Into the *fad diet* group fall all the one food, few food, and crash diets. Here the creativity of the endorsers often borders on the ridiculous. Sometimes the results are tragic.

One woman told me she had eaten nothing but eggs on the first day of her diet. The next day she ate nothing but bananas. The third day she ate nothing but wieners. Then she would start the rotation all over again until she lost the desired amount of weight. At first I thought she was joking, but she was serious. I think her health and emotions might have become seriously damaged had she continued long on that diet.

Weight loss may be very important to you, but it should not be the only factor in choosing a diet. Your body must be properly nourished, or you may lose more than unwanted pounds. Your chosen diet or lifestyle should contribute to your health, not destroy it.

Unless you have only a few pounds to lose and are not really serious about keeping them off over a long period of time, I believe it is best to avoid all fad diets. It is not likely that you will be content to live on grapefruit, grapes, rice, or any extremely limited combination of foods for an extended period of time. The monotony would be unbearable, and your body would suffer from the lack of balanced nutrients needed.

The *low-sugar diets* come under many labels, but all of these are intended to fill the dieter with foods other than sugar, thus reducing calorie intake enough to bring about weight loss. Sugar raises the insulin level in our bodies, and this in turn increases hunger later in the day. The low-sugar foods make it possible to go without refueling for longer periods of time.

For example, a high protein diet could be called a low-sugar diet. Consuming a meal built around meat or cheese, the dieter cuts down on sugar, which reduces calories. This is also true of a diet that depends heavily on complex carbohydrates, and forbids desserts. The discerning dieter will notice that regardless of the name of the diet, the goal is the same: a squeezing out of the high calorie and hunger-producing culprit—sugar.

When I changed my eating habits and stopped using sugar, the pounds began dropping off so fast that I was alarmed, as was my family and even my doctor. I simply had no idea of the amount of other food I would have to eat to make up for the calories I had been taking in through eating sugar-laden treats. When sugar was removed from my diet, my calorie intake plummeted, and so did my weight.

If you decide to use one of the low-sugar diets, be aware that your appetite for sugar is sneaky. Without realizing it, you will find ingenious ways to sweeten your day.

Most people who tell me they don't eat many sweets haven't really thought through their eating habits carefully.

Here a cookie, there a cookie, and there goes the diet.

A friend of mine said it seemed as if the cookie jar whistled at him every time he walked past.

Americans consume mountains of sugar each year, and this sweet saboteur is probably the downfall of more diets than any other food.

Low fat diets are enjoying a good amount of publicity now because of the theory that reducing fat in one's diet cuts down on the chance of getting certain types of cancer. Reducing fat in the diet can also bring about weight loss. Studies show that calories derived from fat are more fattening than those derived from carbohydrates and protein. It seems that the body burns calories to convert carbohydrates and protein into fat for storage, whereas extra fat calories are stored without any calories being burned.[2]

Most other plans for losing weight fall into the *calorie-counting* company. This method of slimming down offers the greatest variety of food and demands the most discipline. Coupled with a good exercise plan, it can be an effective way to lose weight.

Helps for the calorie counter are easily available. Books listing nearly all foods and their calorie content can be found in most bookstores, pharmacies, and food stores. They are well worth the investment.

The American Medical Association says a person leading a moderately active life needs fifteen calories per pound each day. You can find out the approximate number of calories you need to hold your present weight by multiplying your weight times fifteen. This is a general rule, however, because we do not all fit the textbooks when it comes to our rate of calorie burning. Arriving at the correct level of required calories may take some experimenting, but it is possible. If you drop below that level, you should lose weight. Hopefully.

It is generally true that a cut of 500 calories a day will bring about a loss of a pound a week. This takes for granted that you will not reduce your activity level at the same time. You should not go below 1,200 calories a day unless you have been told to do so by your doctor. If you get too lo-cal, you are in danger of depriving your body of necessary vitamins and minerals.

If you choose calorie counting as your way of becoming thin, it will be wise to do so with well-timed and balanced meals.

The Mayo Clinic approach calls for eating the largest meals at breakfast and lunch. This is the time when you will probably be the most active and when your body needs the most calories and nutrients. Fewer calories are needed for your resting time. Eating properly early in the day also reduces appetite and helps prevent overeating at night.[5]

An example of a well-balanced calorie counting diet is one recommended for women by the American Dietetic Association. The diet was presented to clear up confusion created by diet books and claims of single disease diets that are heralded as effective against cancer, osteoporosis, etc. Some guidelines of the diet are as follows:

■ Eat two servings of lean meat daily; four servings of vegetables and fruits; four servings of whole grain breads and cereals.

■ Consume three to four servings daily of low-fat dairy foods or other calcium-rich foods like broccoli, collard greens, and sardines.

■ Get half of your daily calories from carbohydrates like beans, peas, pasta, vegetables, nuts, and seeds.

■ Get no more than a third of calories from fats, and eat a variety: saturated, polyunsaturated, and monosaturated.

■ Eat a variety of fiber-rich foods: fresh fruits with skin, vegetables, beans, and whole grains like brown rice, oat and wheat bran, and oatmeal.

■ Eat iron-rich foods: liver, prunes, kidney and pinto beans, spinach, leafy green vegetables, enriched whole grain breads and cereals.

■ Limit margarine, butter, cooking oils, salad dressings, cookies, cakes, and cream.

■ If dieting, consume ten calories a day for each pound you weigh: 1,400 calories for a 140 pound woman. Don't skip meals.

■ Exercise to control weight and strengthen bones.
■ Limit salt, don't smoke.[4]

Diet Busters

Since the best laid plans of calorie counters can be upset by eating only a few high-caloric foods, I have listed a number of high calorie diet busters for you. A quick look at the list below will show how easily you can pile up calories by eating foods that are packed with them.

DIET BUSTER LIST	CALORIES
Potato chips (10)	114
Pretzels (4 oz.)	442
Soft drink (8 oz.)	96
Chocolate cupcake	205
Almond Joy candy bar	247
Mounds candy bar	274
Chocolate sundae	400
Butterscotch sundae	410
Banana split	1,165
Apple pie (1 piece)	331
Pecan pie (1 piece)	479
Macaroni and cheese (1 cup)	415
Burger King Whopper	630
McDonald's Big Mac	563
Chicken McNuggets and sauce	374
McDonald's Fish Sandwich	432
Pancakes with butter and syrup	500
Granola Bar	110
Peanut Butter Granola Bar	140
French fries (reg. order)	210
Chocolate chip cookie	53
Danish roll	200
Pizza (average piece)	245
Apple Dumpling	345

A Rule to Remember

"A nice lot of information," you say, "but back to the question: Which diet works?"

Any diet will work if it reduces your calorie intake below what you burn in daily activity.

Sound simple?

It is.

But there is one complicating factor: you.

All diets fail without your successful participation. And here you are, discouraged because you have tried before and failed. You've had the best of intentions in the past, to no avail.

No matter.

Past failure in trying to lose weight is no longer a factor.

Take heart.

You've been defeated long enough.

This time is different and the difference is God. He really cares about you and offers all the resources you need to win . . . and lose.

Questions for Application

1. What kind of diets have you tried? How successful have they been?

2. What should you consider when choosing a diet?

3. How can you cope with being on a diet when you eat out? (A quick review of the Diet Buster list may help you answer this question.)

4. What practical dietary guidelines will you establish for yourself today?

4

Those Born Losers

Losing weight is a major undertaking. It involves consuming the flesh and fiber of your own body. And every ounce goes kicking and screaming.

Still, some people lose weight easily. These fast burners can diet for a week and lose more weight than you can in a month. Why?

Research has shown that some overweight people actually eat less than many of their thinner friends but still lose weight more slowly or not at all. The reason for this inequity is simply the difference in metabolism. Some have sluggish metabolisms and burn calories slowly; others have active metabolisms and are able to eat all they want without gaining.

So You're a Hard Loser!

Do you sometimes get so discouraged that you wonder if your metabolism is in reverse? Do you find it easy to gain and hard to lose? Life had been like that for Ron Bushong, and he wrote to tell me about it.

Ron says he had been a fat baby, fat preteen, fat teen, and finally a fat adult. He found himself asking "Why me?" again and again. Let him tell it:

For me, 250 pounds is no problem to attain. Then 300, then 350. It just sneaks up, one bite at a time. A church supper that for many is just a time of good Christian fellowship can, and often did, become an occasion to sin.

I had some success with doctor's diets, weight loss clubs, etc. But it seemed that there was something lacking both in my analyzing the problem and in the solution of it.

My body was a mess! Flat feet, arthritis in my ankles and knees, high blood pressure, heart condition, and high blood sugar. The doctor told me that this situation was going to snowball as long as I was fat.

So, finally I rounded up what remained of my willpower and started on a well-balanced diet. I had lost 10-15 pounds before we traveled to my parents' home on Thanksgiving Day. I was sitting watching TV when my sister came in and threw me a copy of your book, **Weight! A Better Way to Lose.** *I began to read it and couldn't put it down.*

Slowly I realized I had found the missing part to my puzzle. My problem was not just a physical one, nor just an emotional one, but it was a spiritual one!

I finished the book in two sittings.

As a Christian, I realized that God is the victor in spiritual battles. What I had thought of as a curse has really turned out to be a blessing in disguise. It takes daily prayer and meditation to keep the weight off. Every day is a challenge and an opportunity to see God provide every tool I need to fight the battle. I do not win every battle. But I will win the war! Because we have a God who does not know defeat. He strengthens me when I care, and convicts me when I don't.

I have now lost 105 pounds with 30 to go. The arthritis has cleared up. My feet don't hurt. I no longer take blood pressure medicine and I have gone from a 54-inch waist to a 40-inch waist.

Oh, yes, the doctor was motivated to go on a diet also.
God Bless,
Ron Bushong

So there is hope.

Even those who have a natural tendency to be overweight and who have difficulty in losing unwanted pounds can become thin and trim.

Perhaps your constant struggle to lose weight is due to a sluggish metabolism . . . but before you settle on this being your problem be sure to be completely honest about your eating habits.

Remember Achan?

He was the Israelite who stashed some bounty during the conquest of Jericho and failed to report it to Joshua (Josh. 7:16-25). God had told Joshua that all the silver and gold in Jericho was to be consecrated and brought into the treasury of the Lord (Josh. 6:18-19).

Achan saw an expensive garment, two hundred shekels of silver, and a wedge of gold and hid them in his tent, disregarding the commandment of the Lord. As a result, the armies of Israel were defeated in their next battle.

You may have a stash of goodies that no one else knows about. These diet busters are your secret, and you enjoy sneaking off to indulge your appetite for sweets. After all, you deserve a periodic break from the discipline of a diet.

Perhaps. But this kind of catering to your cravings will cancel your gains in self-control.

Don't publicly play the martyr before your quick-loss friends when privately you're not staying with your new lifestyle.

Steps to Stir Up Your Metabolism

You may truly be a slow loser. If so, what can you do about it?

First, consult your doctor. He can order tests that will reveal the nature of your problem. Some deficiency in your body may be the cause of your inability to lose weight.

My wife, Pauline, had found it almost impossible to lose

without reducing calories to dangerous levels until her doctor discovered a low thyroid condition. Under his direction, she began taking thyroid each day to provide a normal amount in her body, and then weight loss became possible for her through healthful dieting and exercise.

The editors of *Prevention Magazine* advocate exercise to fan the flames of a sluggish metabolism. They also suggest eating meals at the same time each day and eating four times a day as a means of perking up your system. For a diet that makes a difference, they recommend eating more complex carbohydrates (fruits, vegetables, and whole grains) while avoiding fats and simple carbohydrates (candy, soft drinks, and desserts).[1]

I believe a positive attitude and a joyful heart combine to speed up metabolism because these make us more active. In losing weight, as in most matters concerning health, "A merry heart doeth good like a medicine: but a broken spirit drieth the bones" (Prov. 17:22).

Breaking the Cycle of Depression

Depression compounds a weight problem. This dark state of mind saps strength and makes self-control difficult. In addition, the depressed person often snacks to get his mind off his problems. Gloom slows him down in all his actions, and he does not burn up energy as he ought.

Since being down keeps your weight up, it is essential to discover the causes of your depression and either conquer or avoid them. The Bible helps us understand some of the dynamics of depression.

You may be depressed because of fear.

Elijah was a prophet of great power. He was courageous and mighty in prayer. On one occasion he raised the dead (1 Kings 17:22), and on another he called down fire from heaven (1 Kings 18:36-38). His rank was such that he appeared with Moses on the Mount of Transfiguration to talk with Jesus about the coming Crucifixion (Matt. 17:3). Many expect him to return to earth in the future as one of the two witnesses spoken of in the Book of Revelation (Rev. 11:3). Still, fear drove him to despair. Threatened by wicked Queen Jezebel, he moaned, "It is enough; now, O Lord, take away my life; for I am not better than my fathers" (1 Kings 19:4).

Like Elijah, you may be defeated by your fears. You sometimes wonder if life is worth living. Your fears concerning your family, your financial security, your health, and the future monopolize your mind.

No wonder you have not been able to control your weight. Your self-discipline is decimated by fear. Everything else is low priority compared to the catastrophes you expect to strike.

What can you do?

You can evaluate your fears.

Of the things you fear, how many are likely to happen to you today? If you can feel safe for the remainder of the day, that is enough for now (Matt. 6:34).

Which of your fears tormented you yesterday? Last week? Last year? Have you been down this road before? How many times have you been troubled by the same thought patterns that paralyze you today, only to find that your expected tragedy never occurred?

What do you fear that is so serious it is not covered by one of the promises found in the Bible? Fear is not new; it is as old as sin (Gen. 3:10). Your fears have not taken God by surprise, and He is able to give you strength enough to rise above them.

Expose your fears to the promises of God. As faith increases, fear decreases. And faith increases as a result of increased daily Bible intake (Rom. 10:17). Perk up your devotional life and see what it does to your fears.

Prayer also conquers fear. Give your fears to the Lord in prayer and refuse to retrieve them. That is what the psalmist did when he was troubled and it worked for him: "I sought the Lord, and He heard me, and delivered me from all my fears" (Ps. 34:4). God still answers prayer. The psalmist's solution will work for you.

You may be depressed because of unconfessed sin.

David had once been known for his merry heart. He was the

singer of sweet songs, the composer of hymns of praise and thanksgiving. In his youth he was so gifted at driving away gloom that King Saul often summoned him to play and sing for him when he was depressed (1 Sam. 16:23).

But David also knew what it was to walk through the valley of despair. He was acquainted with depression. Once he lamented: "I sink in deep mire, where there is no standing: I am come into deep waters, where the floods overflow me. I am weary of my crying: My throat is dried: mine eyes fail while I wait for my God" (Ps. 69:2-3).

What was it that had brought David down? What had stolen his song? He had been unwilling to confess his sins. Read his description of that depressing time: "When I kept silence, my bones waxed old through my roaring all the day long. For day and night Thy hand was heavy upon me: my moisture is turned into the drought of summer" (Ps. 32:2-3).

Thankfully, there is a pleasant ending to David's experience. Finally he could write: "I acknowledged my sin unto Thee, and mine iniquity have I not hid. I said, I will confess my transgressions unto the Lord; and Thou forgavest the iniquity of my sin" (Ps. 32:5).

A wise move for the depressed king. And workable today because, "If we confess our sins, He is faithful and just to forgive us our sins, and to cleanse us from all unrighteousness" (1 John 1:9).

Getting rid of that heavy load of sin you have been carrying could be your key to success in slimming.

You may be depressed because you are hungry.

Some can go without food for long periods of time with little emotional effect. Others cannot.

You may be one who drops into the doldrums when your body runs low on fuel. When that happens, you raid the refrigerator or the snack shelf and blow your diet.

If you feel down when you abstain from food over a long period of time, I suggest you eat when you are hungry. You'll have to avoid high calorie snacks, of course, but there are plenty of nourishing and tasty foods that take away hunger and calm the nerves without adding many calories.

Low fat milk makes a satisfying low calorie snack for me. Skimmed milk is loaded with protein and is not likely to increase your weight. Celery or carrot sticks are favorites of some.

Be creative.

Using your calorie counter's book, you can find a good variety of foods that will boost you over the hungry times and keep you from getting depressed.

Enduring depression to lose weight is not a part of this program. Conquering or avoiding depression is.

You may be depressed because you are overweight.

"Finally," you say, "I wondered how long you would beat around the bush. Every time I look in the mirror, I'm depressed."

Exactly. And that sets up a dreaded cycle. Your weight makes you depressed. You eat high calorie treats because you are depressed, and that increases your weight, causing deeper depression.

Together, we are going to break that cycle.

It can be broken.

One brief statement by author Craig Massey in his article "Pulling Through Depression," has had a continuing positive impact on my life. He says, "While it may be difficult to admit, depression is a deliberate choice."[2]

Undoubtedly, there are some exceptions to Massey's conclusion. Moods can be triggered by physical conditions or mental illnesses, and in these cases more is involved than a decision to be depressed. Nevertheless, his shocking statement has been extremely helpful to me. The thought that I have at times decided to be depressed assures me that I can also decide to come out of that same depression. Finding myself in the pits, I can quickly think back to the experience that caused me to feel depressed and deal with it openly.

"Oh," I say to myself, "I see you've decided to let this get you down." Simply recognizing where I am and why I am there is usually enough to make me chuckle, and by then I am on the road to positive productive living again.

Offering thanksgiving also helps conquer depression.

The moment you begin thanking God for His blessings, however small they may seem in your present frame of mind, you are on your way out of the valley.

When I awake in the morning, knowing that my family members are alive and well, I can count enough blessings to keep me on top of the world all day.

Each morning I thank God that I am alive and that I can see and hear. Looking out a window, I start giving thanks for all the natural beauty that surrounds our home ... and I am grateful daily that we have a home.

Jesus taught His disciples to pray for daily bread. If there is food enough in the house for another meal, it is a day for praising, not for pouting.

Applying the first two verses of Psalm 103 each morning would break the chains of depression for most of us, making us positive people and filling our hearts with the thrill of being alive: "Bless the Lord, O my soul: and all that is within me, bless His holy name. Bless the Lord, O my soul, and forget not all His benefits."

If you find yourself continually depressed despite concentrated effort to stay positive, you may need to receive professional counseling. When you seek out a Christian counselor, fees can almost always be tailored to your budget.

A heavy heart weighs more than you can afford.

Set Realistic Goals

In addition to staying positive and being active, you will be helped by being realistic in your expectations of weight loss and by setting long-range goals.

Don't try to lose fifty pounds by the time of your daughter's wedding or the date of your class reunion.

Success over a long period of time is better than quick losses followed by discouraging gains.

If your family members or classmates cannot accept you as you are, that will be their loss. Your emotional and physical health are more important than making a good impression on others.

"I can only lose a pound a week," a discouraged woman said.

"Well, that's 520 pounds every ten years," I replied.

And the lesson I was trying to get across with a touch of humor is an important one. The real question is not "How many pounds did I lose last week?" but "Have I changed to a lifestyle that is heading toward my long-range goal?"

Goals are important.

My friend Christian Powell had longed to become an attorney. He set this ambitious goal early in life but was afflicted by two dreaded diseases: tuberculosis and polio. Both diseases hospitalized him for long periods of time, and the polio paralyzed most of the major muscles in the lower part of his body. When he was discharged from the hospital after his bout with polio at the age of nineteen, there seemed little hope that he could catch up academically or even go to college, let alone tackle the rigorous and expensive course leading to a law degree.

But Christian was determined to reach his goal and would not concede defeat. Spending many hours each day building up his upper body and studying, he kept pressing toward his goal. One year later, he enrolled in a special college prep course that allowed him to get his high school diploma, and ten years after that he walked across a graduation platform to receive his law degree. By that time, he was married, the father of four sons, and already successful in the field of accounting.

Within a few years after receiving his law degree, Christian was the managing partner in a quickly growing law firm and was active politically and as a land developer. Today, in addition to being involved in several business ventures, he is extremely active in his local church and in a Christian school nearby.

Why has he been so successful?

One of the most important reasons for Christian's success

has been his practice of starting toward distant goals and staying on the course to completion.

Success begins in beginning ... but long-range goals must always be kept in mind. This was Paul's view of life and neither past failures nor present discouragements could keep him from pressing on to his ultimate goal:

> Brethren, I count not myself to have apprehended: but this one thing I do, forgetting those things which are behind, and reaching forth unto those things which are before, I press toward the mark for the prize of the high calling of God in Christ Jesus (Phil. 3:13-14).

While you are heading toward your goal of becoming thin, trim, and triumphant, you will be helped by making much of present victories, no matter how small they may be. Your fast-burning friend may lose seven pounds in seven days while you lose only one, but this should not keep you from celebrating.

A victory is a victory.

Elijah, the prophet, needed only a cloud the size of a man's hand to assure him that God would answer his prayer for rain (1 Kings 18:44). We should follow his example and allow faith to soar at the slightest encouragement.

Setting modest short-range goals will multiply the number of times you feel like a winner and this will make life more enjoyable. In looking to what you want to be in the future, don't miss the joy of today. The psalmist declared: "This is the day which the Lord hath made; we will rejoice and be glad in it" (Ps. 118:24).

Seize each pleasant moment and squeeze out every ounce of joy it contains. The best is yet to come, but don't miss the thrill of being alive right now. Such moment by moment rejoicing contributes to self-discipline and makes ultimate goals attainable.

Fat Fringe Benefits

Your new lifestyle may bring benefits other than weight loss that will provide opportunities to rejoice. Before removing sugar from my diet, I had problems with blurred vision. Thinking my sight was getting poorer with age, I went for an eye examination, but the exam revealed little change and no good reason for the blurring. After I stopped eating sweets, the blurring ceased and has not returned.

Debbie Girgenti, who attends a weight loss class where members use *Weight! A Better Way to Lose*, had a similar experience. Her family has a history of eye problems and when she began having difficulty with her left eye, she feared this family condition might be coming upon her. A consultation with her eye doctor added to her concern when he said they would just have to wait and see what developed.

Meanwhile, Debbie had gained thirty pounds and as a result, started attending a Christian diet class to get her weight under control. Soon she was losing pounds and inches and feeling great.

When she went for her next eye examination, the doctor asked Debbie what changes she had made in her life. Then, while she was pondering his question, he followed with another: "Have you been on a diet?"

After hearing Debbie's description of her new eating habits, the doctor explained that a good diet is not a cure for everything, but that in her case it had cleared up the problem in her left eye. Her eyes are now healthier than when her diet had been out of control, and she is enjoying one of the fringe benefits of her new lifestyle.

Barbara King, a pastor's wife and homemaker was experiencing extreme fatigue. Her many duties in the church and at home kept her drained of energy. Then she began attending a Christian diet group and applying biblical principles of weight control. Soon she found her strength returning. While losing unwanted pounds, she gained new energy. She writes:

I am moving toward my goal of twenty pounds. I have energy and feel so much better in the short time of three months. The Lord has even helped me resist rich foods during the Christmas holiday season. The Lord is truly helping me to delight to do His will. Praise the Lord.

Two Vital Ingredients in Slimming Success

So, you can become thin and trim, even if your metabolism is not as rapid as the metabolism of your friends who lose weight so easily. But it will be important to remember that a positive attitude and regular exercise are vital to success.

Reject negative thinking.

Choose Paul's thought patterns for your own:

> Finally, brethren, whatsoever things are true, whatsoever things are honest, whatsoever things are just, whatsoever things are pure, whatsoever things are lovely, whatsoever things are of good report; if there be any virtue, and if there be any praise, think on these things (Phil. 4:8).

Expect to achieve the weight you desire; to become the person you want to be in the will of God. Expectation is an important part of faith, and it is through faith that all of God's gifts are given.

Get a spring in your step that reflects your new outlook on life, and if you do not increase your intake of food, it must make a difference in your weight. At the University of California, Dr. Grant Gwinup studied a group of overweight women who took a brisk, half-hour walk every day for a year. Each woman lost an average of twenty-two pounds. Their range of loss was from ten to thirty-eight pounds.

Rise earlier.
Attempt more.
Savor life.
Come alive.

Change your attitude about eating. Make meal time more than fill-up-time. Enjoy the people around your table. Delight in each delicious mouthful of food. Determine to make your meal last longer without eating more. Take smaller bites so that you will not finish so quickly.

Give thanks each day that you have a slower metabolism than some and that this demands more discipline and activity to achieve goals in weight control. Those quick weight loss people can lose without much effort; therefore, they miss out on the thrill of accomplishment through self-control and active living.

You have the greater challenge.

Accept that challenge and expect to meet it in the power of Christ. That's what abundant living is all about.

Questions for Application

1. What do you think about Craig Massey's statement: "Depression is a deliberate choice"?

2. Describe the characteristics of a person you know who has a merry heart. How has a merry heart helped this person?

3. Think of a time when you were depressed. How did you escape the feeling of depression? Based on your reading of this chapter, how will you handle depression differently now?

4. What short-range goal can you establish for exercise and developing a positive attitude? What are your long-range goals for exercise and developing a positive attitude?

5

The Devil and Your Diet

Does the devil want you fat?
My answer to this question seems to intrigue talk show producers and hosts and hostesses more than any other aspect of my approach of losing weight the Bible way. Their interest in this dimension of Christian weight control is not surprising since most other approaches give no thought to the spiritual battle involved in losing weight. Interviewers find the concept of satanic opposition to becoming thin and trim hard to swallow. They are also usually unaware of the promise of victory over our enemy through the power of Christ.

Satan's Strategy

A look at Satan's past strategies should clear up any doubt about his interest in blocking your effort to improve your life through Spirit-directed weight control. His aim has always been our destruction, and he is not above using our lack of self-control in eating to reach his goal.

Mankind's first temptation involved food (Gen. 3:1-7). Our first parents were allowed to eat anything in the Garden of

Eden except the fruit of one tree. This generous arrangement
provided them with immense variety. They should therefore
have had little trouble avoiding the forbidden fruit. Yet Satan
was able to turn Eve's attention away from all that God had
given them to focus on the one restriction.

Many diets die from obsession with a restriction. One slice
of devil's food cake (well-named) becomes more important
than pounds of peace of mind. Truckloads of nourishing food
cannot compete with one delicious dessert. Self-control fails.
One bite can begin a sugar binge, and when that happens, all
is lost . . . except weight.

The real purpose of our enemy in the Garden of Eden, of
course, was to bring about the fall of mankind, resulting in
lasting destructive effects upon God's creation. A study of the
Bible reveals a continuing satanic effort to turn people away
from God and to injure or destroy their bodies, which are
such an important evidence of God's creative work.

Job was both healthy and wealthy before his encounter with
the devil. As a result of Satan's attack, this good man lost
everything, including his health. The origin of Job's suffering is
revealed in Job 2:7: "So went Satan forth from the presence of
the Lord, and smote Job with sore boils from the sole of his
foot unto his crown." How the devil delighted in robbing this
man of his health.

Other accounts of bodily injury or illness caused by satanic
power are recorded in the New Testament. A typical case is
the one Jesus and the disciples encountered after they had
descended from the Mountain of Transfiguration. They met a
desperate father who begged them to help his son.

Dr. Luke explains the meeting as follows:

> And, behold, a man of the company cried out, saying,
> "Master, I beseech thee, look upon my son: for he is
> mine only child. And, lo, a spirit taketh him, and he
> suddenly crieth out; and it teareth him that he foameth
> again, and bruising him hardly departeth from him"
> (Luke 9:38-39).

Clearly, we face a cruel enemy who is bent on our destruction and pleased with our misery. Jesus summarized Satan's purpose in all of our lives: "The thief cometh not, but for to steal, and to kill, and to destroy" (John 10:10).

He may kill with calories.

Don't cooperate with him.

Losses When You Gain

If you still doubt that the devil wants to keep you overweight, consider what he gains when you stuff yourself with food.

Your intemperance makes you disobedient to the Word of God. Solomon warned: "Be not among winebibbers; among riotous eaters of flesh: For the drunkard and the glutton shall come to poverty" (Prov. 23:20-21).

Overeating is one of the more respectable sins among believers. Some Christians even boast of their great capacity for food, not remembering that drunkards and gluttons are relegated to the same company in the Scriptures.

The devil delights when emotional hang-ups that come from being overweight hinder your Christian service. You may feel self-conscious about being in front of crowds because you are not happy with your appearance. You lack confidence, so you withdraw from people. You are no longer active in your church. Your gifts and talents are not used as God intended them to be.

The devil has you where he wants you ... sitting on the sidelines instead of being active in serving your Lord.

By limiting your Christian service and stifling your potential, you become inactive and make it that much easier to gain weight. This is another of the discouraging cycles of obesity, a cycle you can conquer in the power of Christ.

Then there is the stewardship of your money and possessions. Satan is interested in keeping your material resources from their highest purpose—investment in the ministry of Christ around the world.

Obesity is expensive.

Believe it or not, each calorie that contributed to your overweight condition cost something. "There is no such thing as a free lunch." You bought your bulges.

Also, you have probably spent a considerable amount of money trying to get rid of your extra weight. Diet pills, doctor's advice, exercise club memberships, and uncounted magazines and books containing weight control help have all been part of the expense of being overweight and trying to lose pounds.

Don't you think it's time to cut the fat out of your budget?

One woman who became concerned about the amount of money she had wasted on food and trying to lose decided to do something about it. She started cutting out snacks and sweets, and she deposited the cost of that food in a fund to be given to the Lord's work. Imagine her double delight as she saw the fund growing and her fat going.

The issue of Christian stewardship is a biblical one and has long been stressed in areas of life other than weight loss. But what about all those calorie rich goodies that seem to be a must at every gathering for fellowship? How much of that waste becomes waist? If we were to cash in our calories, how many would it take to support a missionary? Satan must smile at our double standards.

Satan must also be delighted when we go on in our self-satisfied way, feeding ourselves but ignoring those who are hungry.

Many are hungry today. What a great impact the message of salvation would have for the needy if we delivered the Gospel with the compassion Jesus demonstrated. You can be sure that Satan does not want this kind of outpouring of love to take place.

Think about this: you can transfer those unwanted pounds of yours to some starving frame. You can give those extra calories you've been consuming to people who need them. If you do not know any hungry people, missionary relief organizations within the mail-reach of every Christian will be delighted to assist you in your pound exchange project. You may be far more creative in developing this area of stewardship than I have been in making suggestions. I hope so and would be pleased to hear about your pound-transfer program and its success.

It should be clear by now that you can expect satanic opposition as you make an effort to get in shape. Let's summarize the reasons:
1. The devil wants you to live in a way that will ruin your health and shorten your life.
2. The devil wants you to disobey God's Word and lack self-control.
3. The devil wants to keep you from Christian service.
4. The devil wants to sidetrack you from Christian stewardship.

Resources in Christ to Overcome Satan

Since the devil wants to keep you fat, how can you ever hope to achieve your goal of becoming thin and trim?

There is but one answer. You must tap the resources available to you in Christ. Satan is too strong an enemy for you to face alone. If you confront him alone, you are sure to lose . . . and gain.

F.B. Meyer wrote:

> There is only one way by which the tempter·can be met. He laughs at our good resolutions and ridicules the pledges with which we fortify ourselves. There is only One whom he fears; One who in the hour of greatest weakness conquered him; and who has been raised far above all principality and power, that He may succor and deliver all frail and tempted souls.[1]

Do you feel frail when tempted? Then follow God's formula for victory: "Submit yourselves therefore to God. Resist the devil, and he will flee from you" (James 4:7). Submit to God and resist the devil. Upon doing so, you will win over your enemy. God guarantees that Satan will flee from you. Victory will be yours . . . every time.

Steve Main, one of the directors of Roger Campbell Ministries, needed to lose forty pounds. His weight had been up and down the scales before, but now he wanted to tune his body to a point of new vigor and health that would enable him to keep his busy schedule without feeling drained every day.

His plan called for cutting out some of his favorite foods: most bread, red meat, salt, and desserts. He said he intended to leave something on his plate at the end of each meal.

But this was no easy task. Steve had been a hearty eater. Refusing such things as snacks on frequent plane trips and cutting calories enough in other ways to get trim presented a real challenge.

One secret of Steve's success was keeping up his daily devotional time. The added strength he gained from daily Bible reading and prayer proved to be enough to enable him to lose the desired amount.

What was he doing?

Drawing upon the power of Christ to overcome temptation.

As the pounds dropped off, Steve found that one victory led to another. Compliments by family members and friends encouraged him as did the opportunity of wearing new clothes in the sizes he had set as his goals. He feels good about his accomplishment but knows he could not have achieved it so readily without using the spiritual resources available to him to overcome temptation.

The Bible is a powerful resource to use when tempted. I suggest memorizing certain verses that apply to winning over temptation when you are trying to lose weight.

The psalmist says the Bible can keep us clean and give continual victory over temptation: "Wherewithal shall a young man cleanse his way? By taking heed thereto according to Thy Word. Thy Word have I hid in my heart, that I might not sin against Thee" (Ps. 119:9-11).

The Bible on the coffee table will not enable you to win over temptation. According to the psalmist, it is the Word of God in our hearts that makes us victorious.

So the Bible must be part of life. This means reading it daily and applying its truth in everyday situations. I find it helpful to write out Bible verses on cards daily and keep them on my desk or carry them with me.

You may find another method of taking God's Word into your heart that works better for you. Whatever method you chose, be sure that you are systematically taking the Bible into your mind so that it can find its way to your heart and do its part to enable you to win over temptation.

The Sameness of Temptation

One of the encouraging things about temptation is its universal sameness. Every temptation that comes our way has been experienced by someone else. The setting may have changed, but the basic temptation is unchanged. We are all tempted by "the lust of the flesh, the lust of the eyes, and the pride of life" (1 John 2:15-16).

Consider the temptation of Eve again:

> And when the woman saw that the tree was good for food, and that it was pleasant to the eyes, and a tree to be desired to make one wise, she took of the fruit thereof, and did eat, and gave also unto her husband with her; and he did eat (Gen. 3:6).

The fruit would taste good (the lust of the flesh); it was pleasant to the eyes (the lust of the eyes); it would make one wise (the pride of life). This is not to say that all things that taste and look good are sinful. But this fruit had been expressly forbidden by the Lord. These characteristics then became the tools of the tempter, causing Eve to fall.

That first temptation of Jesus also had to do with food, as was the case in the temptation of Eve. Eve was tempted when surrounded by an abundance of delicious food that she was allowed to eat. Our Lord, on the other hand, was tempted after He had been fasting for forty days in a barren wilderness:

> Then was Jesus led up by the Spirit into the wilderness to

be tempted of the devil. And when He had fasted forty days and forty nights, He was afterward an hungered. And when the tempter came to Him, he said, If Thou be the Son of God, command that these stones be made bread (Matt. 4:1-3).

Dr. John R. Rice has written:

"Why did Jesus fast forty days? So that He might be as weak as any man ever would be when tempted. He was as hungry, as frail; the temptation as overpowering as any human being ever faced.

"Was Jesus really tempted? Did He feel the tug and pull of desire? The answer is that He most certainly was tempted. The Scripture says so. He was hungry, tomentingly, fiercely hungry! His poor stomach gnawed with desire. His weakened body cried out for food, and He doubtless felt all the lightheadedness and perhaps delirium that men who go long days without food feel. Certainly, here was a real and definite temptation, as definite and real as any man ever faced. Jesus never one time gave way to it, but He felt the pull of every other temptation that men are ever tempted with. His body was like our bodies. He put himself in our place and yet never sinned."[2]

There in that barren place, tempted to change stones into bread (a miracle that was well within His power), Jesus answered the tempter: "It is written, 'Man shall not live by bread alone, but by every word that proceedeth out of the mouth of God'" (Matt. 4:4).

Are you wrestling with temptation because you are hungry? The next time you are tempted to eat something that will add too many calories to your day, remember the temptation of Jesus.

Because He overcame the desire to eat when hungry, you can too. His power is made available to you through faith, and you do not have to yield to temptation.

Limits on Temptation

Another source of encouragement for the calorie-counter is revealed in 1 Corinthians 10:13:

> There hath no temptation taken you but such as is common to man: but God is faithful, who will not suffer you to be tempted above that ye are able; but will with the temptation also make a way to escape, that ye may be able to bear it.

What a promise!

No temptation that is beyond your ability to resist will ever be allowed to come your way.

In order to make such a guarantee, God has to know the limit of your strength. And He does! He has already measured your breaking point and forbids any temptation to go beyond it. Our strengths and weaknesses are well-known to Him. The psalmist wrote: "For He knoweth our frame; He remembereth that we are dust" (Ps. 103:14).

Neither trials nor temptations can move beyond the limit placed upon them by our faithful God. Henry Ward Beecher said, "No physician ever weighed out medicine to his patients with half so much care and exactness as God weighs out to us every trial. Not one grain too much does He ever permit to be put on the scale."[3]

Shortly after I was told to stop eating sugar, we were being entertained by friends, and I was offered a piece of pie made with an artificial sweetener. Not being sure if this would be safe for me to eat, I declined. I asked my doctor about the use of sugar substitutes at my next visit to his office.

"Ah, you don't need them," he replied.

That's easy for him to say, I thought.

But now I am glad he gave that advice for it taught me to face the temptation to compromise my diet and overcome it. Since God has limited all of my temptations to what I can overcome, I am able to successfully resist the temptation to eat desserts.

Bring on the strawberry shortcake piled high with whipped cream. I can pass it by.

Serve those honey glazed raised donuts that used to be my midmorning delight, and I will politely refuse them.

Take me into your town's most tempting bakery and ask me to gaze at some of the delicious creations, and I'll still not be moved.

How do I know?

I've been there and won.

"You must have great willpower," someone says.

Not at all.

I've simply learned that as a Christian I am equipped to win over temptation and that my Heavenly Father has set limits on the tempter and all temptation.

In His wisdom, God has required that every temptation we face be accompanied by a way of escape. These disaster exits may take many forms, but they all offer ways to freedom.

Sometimes other people have been God's way of escape. Remembering the consistent lifestyle of another has on occasion been enough to deliver tempted ones to safety. The arrival of another Christian right on time has frequently been just what someone needed to keep from yielding to temptation in despair.

So many people in my home area are acquainted with my biblical approach to weight control that when I walk into a restaurant, I have sometimes caused diners to change their orders. Convicted customers have told me that seeing me there has reminded them that they do not have to yield to the temptation to eat high calorie foods and begin a trip into bondage again. Although this situation has usually been explained to me in a humorous manner, the incident clearly illustrates an important element of truth.

Diversions of various kinds have delivered those who were tempted. Perhaps you remember a time when something unexpected turned your mind from some enticement at the crucial moment to keep you from yielding to temptation. If so, thank God for His faithfulness in providing a way of escape for you.

We Are Equipped to Win
When it comes to temptation, then, we are all without excuse. God has limited both the tempter and temptation to what others have endured and to what we can overcome. He is faithful and has equipped us with the power to win every contest.

Commenting on God's provision for Christians to conquer temptation, Dr. M.R. DeHaan, founder of the Radio Bible Class, wrote: "And this brings us to the glorious truth of the grace of God, which can enable us to live above the circumstances of life, and not be defeated, but victorious in all that we do. We need not fall short of victory."[4]

The good doctor said it well: When tempted, we can win.

We must be on guard continually, remembering that we face a formidable foe. He knows our weaknesses and is quick to attack us where we are most vulnerable. But we are not destined for defeat. The Holy Spirit lives within us and is greater in power than our enemy: "Ye are of God, little children, and have overcome them: because greater is He that is in you, than he that is in the world" (1 John 4:4).

Our Saviour defeated Satan at the cross. His death and resurrection provide complete victory when we appropriate His power by faith. Through total submission to God and determined resistance to Satan, we *can* overcome the one who seeks our defeat.

Sharing concepts to overcome Satan in his book *Satan's Angels,* Ken Anderson wrote:

The closer a Christian walks with his Lord, the more conscious he will become of satanic interference. In my own experiences, I have come to often say to myself, "Well, there he is again." Invariably when God gives me a special opportunity to serve Him, Satan

appears on the scene. But no matter! Through the
simple exercise of faith, I have authority over Satan![5]

That same authority is available to every Christian and has
become a part of my prayer life every day. Awesome as the
power of Satan may be, we need not fear. Our Lord will
shelter us in His love, arm us for every conflict, and enable us
to win.

Since it is vital that we win in this spiritual battle, it is
important to understand that God has provided exactly what
we need for the battle. In addition to giving us His strength to
compensate for our weakness, He has given us equipment
with which to fight against the powers of darkness. Paul calls
this the "armor of God" and urges us to make full use of it.
You will find this armor for Christian soldiers described in
Ephesians 6:14-18. I suggest that you give some time to the
study of this important text.

Finally, don't forget to make full use of the power of prayer.
When the going gets tough and you feel like you're going to
give in to the enemy, remember that God answers prayer. His
ear is always open to your call. He's never out to lunch and
takes no refreshment breaks. You can pray without ceasing,
and He will never tire of hearing from you.

Martin Luther was once passing through a severe trial and
feeling depressed. The struggle against the enemy seemed too
much for him.

Sensing his despair, his wife dressed in black and entered his
study saying: "God is dead!"

"Nonsense, woman, God lives!" answered Luther.

"If you believe that God is living, act like it! Live like it!" she
replied.[6]

Let us face every battle with our enemy believing that our
living Lord really cares and that He will bring us through to
victory. That is His promise to all who trust Him. We can
claim His power to overcome, even in this very personal area
of our lives: becoming thin and trim and better able to serve
Him.

Questions For Application

1. Review the list on page 67 of reasons why Satan wants you fat. What other reasons can you add to this list?

2. Think of a time when you were tempted (perhaps to over-eat). How did you handle the temptation?

3. During an average day, do you notice a time period when you are often tempted to overeat? What can you do to avoid giving in to this temptation?

6

Faith Can Move That Moutain

> How were you eating at the time you looked like that? Do you have faith to believe you can first a patter to dendly + you can always look like that?

"**D**o you recognize me?" asked a woman who approached me after I had ministered in a service at her church.

"I know I should," I replied, embarrassed that I could not call her name to mind.

"I've lost ninety pounds since you were here last year," she continued.

No wonder I didn't recognize her.

What had made her success possible?

Faith in God.

In believing, she had found the joy and discipline needed to lose weight, and now she was clearly delighted with her achievement.

Many others have shared her discovery.

Charlie Shedd's Big Surrender

Charlie Shedd had tried and failed to lose weight many times, but there came a time when a new start, grounded in faith, changed his life and led to successful weight control. He wrote:

Fifteen years and one hundred twenty pounds ago, I dropped to my knees and prayed: "Lord, I've tried for years to whip this problem of obesity. I've been on banana diets and eaten red meat. I've taken pills and bought reducing belts. I've read books, attended lectures, joined clubs, enrolled in courses. But I'm still fat. I weigh too much. And I need help. In the Good Book You promise if anyone has enough faith he can say to a mountain, 'Go away,' and it will go. There's a mountain of flesh on me. I've been trying to move it ever since I was a boy. I've been laughed at. I've been ridiculed. I've rationalized. I've lied. I've had times when I cared and times when I didn't.

"I've decided to quit and promised I'd be good. Then we were invited out, and this woman makes the best biscuits. I've sworn off, and before I knew it, I found myself sitting at the fountain lapping a milkshake.

"Now I mean business. I accept You at Your word. Today I say to this mountain, 'Get moving.' I have faith that the two of us can move it together. This is the big surrender. I'm turning my body over to You once and for all. I can't manage it alone. From this day on, I'll eat what You tell me to eat and live how You want me to live. Amen."[1]

Shedd shed his extra weight with a lifestyle anchored in faith. So can you.

The Key to Successful Living

We should not be surprised to discover that faith exercised in daily life is the key to successful living. Eternal life comes through faith in Jesus Christ, and this same faith makes the abundant life that He promised a reality here and now (John 10:10). C.H. Spurgeon observed: "A little faith will bring your soul to heaven, but great faith will bring heaven to your soul."

We are saved by faith (Eph. 2:8-9), but that is only the

beginning. "The just shall live by faith" (Heb. 10:38).

That verse caught fire in Martin Luther's heart and sparked the Reformation. It shaped the world. Faith, then, must be powerful enough to help you get in shape.

Dr. V. Raymond Edman, former president and late chancellor of Wheaton (IL) College, said:

> Faith is dead to doubts, dumb to impossibilities, knows nothing but success. Faith lifts its hands up through the threatening clouds, lays hold of Him who has all power in heaven and on earth. Faith makes the uplook good, the outlook bright, the inlook favorable, and the future glorious.[2]

Faith Adds a New Dimension

Does this mean that faith will zap off those extra pounds overnight?

Not quite. It does mean that you will tackle your problem and launch this effort with absolute confidence that you will win this time. Faith adds a new dimension when you face difficulties. Old failures no longer demand present defeat.

Great faith is built on the conviction that God can do anything. Most Christians believe this but do not act upon it. They accept omnipotence intellectually, but this belief makes little difference in their lives. Consequently, problems loom large, burdens become heavy, and the future becomes something to be feared.

Most of us need the challenge given to Jeremiah: "Behold, I am the LORD, the God of all flesh: is there anything too hard for me?" (Jer. 32:27)

J. Hudson Taylor, the famous missionary, wrote:

> Many Christians estimate difficulties in the light of their own resources, and thus attempt little and often fail in the little they attempt. All God's giants have been weak men who did great things for God because they reckoned on His power and presence with them.[3]

When my beloved wife, Pauline, entered the hospital, we thought she had a severe case of flu. We discovered that instead of the flu, she had been stricken with a life-threatening condition. For reasons still unknown, her blood had begun to destroy itself. Our doctor explained that she had become allergic to her own blood.

After receiving word of the seriousness of Pauline's condition, I returned from the hospital and walked through our home, praying as I walked. Evidences of her loving work were everywhere: the pictures on the walls, the arrangement of the furniture, decorations of her own making. Her special touch was upon everything. My heart was heavy, and by the time I had finished my prayer tour, hot tears were burning trenches in my face.

Just at that point, the back door opened and our oldest son, David, entered the house. Seeing my tears, he put his arms around me, saying, "Don't worry, Dad. We're praying and everything will be fine. Have faith."

Faith.

How I needed it!

I had been with others many times when the lives of their loved ones were on the line and had encouraged them to believe, but this was different. It was one thing to exhort someone in distress and another to experience it yourself.

During the difficult days that followed, I was moved by the promise of the power of faith given in Matthew 17:20: "If ye have faith as a grain of mustard seed, ye shall say unto this mountain, 'remove hence to yonder place'; and it shall remove; and nothing shall be impossible unto you." This verse both challenged me and imparted hope. I longed to plumb its depths and harness its power.

I deeply appreciated the efforts of the doctors during this crisis, but apart from giving steroids and blood transfusions to sustain life, there seemed little that could be done.

Faith offered another dimension for hope and brought a break in the clouds. I prayed earnestly and hundreds of others prayed with me.

① Eating healthy is smart —
② Small portions are satisfying +
all of my body requires

Then came an encouraging phone call from our family doctor. He had thoughtfully instructed the person placing the call to immediately assure me that this call from his office was not to bring bad news. When he was finally on the line, the doctor's first words were, "Whatever you're doing, keep doing it!" Pauline's blood count was beginning to rise.

Many, many good years have passed since that crisis, and Pauline has had no recurrence of the problem that had brought her to death's door. Our mountain has been removed, and I am confident that faith in the hearts of praying people moved it.

A friend of mine, a missionary, entered a local hospital for surgery. After opening him up, however, the doctors found him to be filled with cancer. He was sent home and told he had about six months to live.

This man of faith and his wife settled on a Bible verse as an anchor of hope during those difficult days. It was Philippians 1:20: "So now also Christ shall be magnified in my body, whether it be by life, or by death."

My friend related this experience to me *fourteen* years after he had been sent home to die. At our last contact, he was headed for another mission field to serve his Lord.

The New Testament abounds with miracles and promises that confirm the limitless power of God. One of the greatest of these miracles is the incarnation of Jesus Christ. When the Angel Gabriel appeared to Mary with the message that she would bear a son and that He would be called the Son of the Highest, she couldn't understand it. In fact, she questioned: "How shall this be, seeing I know not a man?" (Luke 1:34) The angel assured Mary that with God, nothing is impossible (Luke 1:37).

That exciting promise is for you too.

You can become thin and trim. Your past failures are not a factor because with God nothing shall be impossible. He will give you the discipline you need and will guide you in developing an active lifestyle that will enable you to reach your goal.

Faith-building Bible Study

Faith is developed by exposure to the Bible. It cannot be pumped up or faked. Its source is the Scriptures: "So then faith cometh by hearing, and hearing by the word of God" (Rom. 10:17).

God's promises encourage faith. As you take time to study the Bible, you will find guarantees of strength, peace, courage, salvation, power, victory, and answered prayer. You will read of the exploits of others who have conquered through faith. As you identify with these promises and personal triumphs, your faith will increase. Depression will depart. Expectation will emerge.

I set no quotas for speed in getting through the Bible or even a book of the Bible. I may read several chapters or only a few. In Bible reading for devotional purposes, quality reading is far more important than getting a great number of chapters read.

I am searching for faith-building Bible verses that will equip me for whatever should come my way. I expect these promises from God to keep me on course and bolster my faith for anything my day may hold.

Now there will be days when we don't feel like reading the Bible. What shall we do then?

George Müller wrote:

> It is a common temptation of Satan to make us give up the reading of the Word and prayer when our enjoyment is gone; as if it were no use to read the Scriptures when we do not enjoy them, and as if it were no use to pray when we have no spirit of prayer. The truth is that, in order to enjoy the Word, we ought to continue to read it, and the way to obtain a spirit of prayer is to continue praying. The less we read the Word of God, the less we desire to read it, and the less we pray, the less we desire to pray.[4]

A simple way of handling such dry times for me is to decide

not to feed my body until I have fed my soul. A healthy morning appetite will then halt neglect of the Bible in a hurry, bringing the blessing of beginning the day with nourishment of the soul and the joy of giving priority to self-control.

Many starve themselves spiritually by neglecting the Bible and are therefore too weak to overcome temptation and enjoy the abundant life. One of the teachers, developed in our first classes on weight control, said she had learned that building up the inner person was absolutely necessary if she was to trim down the outer person.

Praying in Faith

I believe it is best to have a quiet time with the Lord in the morning, unless your schedule demands a different time of the day. Rising a bit earlier for Bible reading and prayer is a great way to start the day, recharging you before facing the responsibilities of the workplace or the home.

I begin my morning devotions with an enriching time of thanksgiving. Following this comes prayer, which includes confession of sin and asking in faith for God to supply my needs and grant the desires of my heart.

Some wonder if it is proper to ask God for the desires of our hearts. Numerous promises in the Bible assure us that God will answer our prayers for the things we need and want: "Call unto me, and I will answer thee, and show thee great and mighty things, which thou knowest not" (Jer. 33:3). Another favorite promise of many is Psalm 37:4: "Delight thyself also in the Lord; and He shall give thee the desires of thine heart."

I am grateful for those who have come into my life and taught me how to pray in faith. In one church where I was the pastor, the custodians were people of great faith and deep devotion to the Lord. Often, this couple would spend time praying with me in my study for the needs of the church and other concerns.

How fervently this husband and wife prayed! They asked God for things I didn't even know He had in stock. And they believed He would answer. Their faith was contagious and it enriched mine. Soon I found myself becoming bolder in prayer and more likely to expect God to answer.

How bold are your prayers?

Do you expect God to answer?

According to the Bible, there are only two limits on prayer: we should not ask for things which we consume on our lusts (James 4:3), and we should not ask for anything outside the will of God (1 John 5:14). Neither of these restrictions should keep us from praying for success in losing weight. So . . . pray about reaching your goal in weight control.

Prayer can bring victory to losers; success to those who would otherwise fail. It makes cowards courageous and often brings hope even to those given to the dark clouds of depression. Prayer can even bring discipline to the dinner table and the power to choose exercise over an easy chair.

But some do not pray in faith. They mouth words but do not expect God to come through for them. Contrasting real faith with what he called "pseudo faith," A.W. Tozer wrote:

> Pseudo faith always arranges a way out to serve in case God fails it. Real faith knows only one way and gladly allows itself to be stripped of any second way or make-shift substitutes. For true faith, it is either God or total collapse. And not since Adam first stood up on earth has God failed a single man or woman who trusted Him.[5]

Does God answer prayer?

Ask David, who wrote: "This poor man cried, and the Lord heard him, and saved him out of all his troubles" (Ps. 34:6).

Ask Daniel, who spent a night with a den full of hungry lions and lived to tell about it (Dan. 6).

Ask Jonah, who cried out to God from inside the great fish and soon found himself on dry ground, being commissioned again to serve his Lord (Jonah 2–3).

Ask Peter, who was delivered from prison by an angel in answer to the prayers of the early church (Acts 12).

But we must be careful not to limit the power of prayer to Bible times. Prayer is the key to victory in every area of life, and praying in faith will be vital to your success in becoming thin and trim. This kind of practical praying will bring new hope, even if you have tried to lose before and failed.

Faith Grows through Exercise

Acting in faith will also be important to faith's development. Like most things, faith grows with exercise.

David was able to face the giant, Goliath, because he had *already* conquered wild beasts that had attacked his father's sheep. By the time Moses lifted his rod and parted the Red Sea, he had *already* witnessed the power of God in bringing the plagues upon Egypt.

To quote George Müller again:

> Some may say, "Oh, I shall never have the gift of faith Mr. Müller has got." This is a mistake—it is the greatest error—there is not a particle of truth in it. My faith is the same kind of faith that all of God's children have had. It is the same kind that Simon Peter had, and all Christians may obtain like faith. My faith is their faith, though there may be more of it because my faith has been a little more developed by exercise than theirs; but their faith is precisely the faith that I exercise, only with regard to degree, mine may be more strongly exercised.[6]

If you want to increase your faith, you must start using the faith you now have. Exercising faith can take many forms of expression. Perhaps you will want to increase your giving to your church, trusting the Lord to meet all of your personal needs. This would be an act of faith based on promises of provision given in the Bible such as Proverbs 3:9-10, Malachi 3:10, Luke 6:38, to name a few.

Whatever you do in faith will add adventure to life. As God honors your faith with answers to your prayers, your faith will grow even more. It is a blessed cycle and one that is too often neglected by believers.

Those who watch unwanted pounds drop off as a result of their new way of living are always thrilled to have discovered an answer to their weight problem that is both effective and exciting. Best of all, embarking on this unique weight-loss adventure has a positive effect on all other areas of their lives.

God Can Do Anything

A Roman army officer came to Jesus, seeking help for his servant who was sick of the palsy and in great pain. Jesus assured him that He would come to his house and heal his servant. Upon hearing the Lord's promise, the officer replied:

> "Lord, I am not worthy that Thou shouldest come under my roof: but speak the word only, and my servant shall be healed. For I am a man under authority, having soldiers under me; and I say to this man, Go, and he goeth; and to another, Come, and he cometh; and to my servant, do this, and he doeth it" (Matt. 8:8-9).

The Lord was moved by this officer's complete confidence in Him, saying, "I have not found so great faith, no not in Israel" (Matt. 8:10).

The officer's faith was declared great because he believed that the power of Christ was great enough to meet his need. He saw no limit to our Lord's ability to respond to his request. His simple trust in the power of Christ amounted to great faith. As a result of his faith, his servant was healed.

Our faith grows in direct proportion to our confidence that God can do anything, and He can! Jeremiah wrote: "Ah Lord God! behold, Thou hast made the heaven and the earth by Thy great power and stretched out arm, and there is nothing too hard for Thee" (Jer. 32:17).

So, trust God to enable you to become thin and trim, to make it possible for you to lose those troublesome pounds that drain your strength and injure your health. Tell your friends and family members that you are going to work on losing weight and gaining the appearance that you have wanted for so long. Let it be known that you are trusting the Lord to give you the courage and discipline necessary to reach your goal.

Refuse to consider failure. Remember, you are acting in faith. And God rewards faith. Think, then, only of success.

Reject negative thinking.

Doubt the doubters.

There are some who are sure to doubt your ability to meet your goal. They will point to all of those other times in the past when you have had good intentions and failed. They will tell you it isn't worth the effort. A few will bring you gifts of your favorite foods, hoping to sabotage your diet. Others will have genuine concern for you in this struggle and will urge you to forget the whole thing so that you are not under any special pressure to succeed.

Lovingly tune them out.

You have too much to lose by not losing. Your health, your happiness, and your future are weighed each time you step on the scales.

Besides, you do not have to be fat.

Faith can move that mountain.

Questions for Application

1. If your name were listed with the faithful saints in Hebrews 11, how would your faith be described?

2. Think back over the week. How much time have you spent in faith-building Bible study and prayer? How has this affected your ability to resist temptation?

3. What step of faith will you take in the week ahead?

Faith in God to assist in prayer & continued exercise for myself
10-2-06

7

Get That Moutain Moving

Y ou've heard it before:
"The most important exercise in losing weight is pushing yourself away from the table."

That subtle half-truth implies that physical exercise isn't all that important to weight loss. But it is!

I am married to a lady who keeps herself in shape. She disciplines her body and stays trim. For more than thirty years, an exercise program has been an important part of her life. Without her example, this book would not have been written.

Why Exercise Is Important
Reducing our intake of calories is one way to lose weight. The most satisfying and effective way to lose, however, is by both cutting down on calories and increasing exercise. For long-range success, both of these approaches should be built into a permanent lifestyle change.

Some Christians quote the Bible as a cop-out on added exercise. Their favorite verse is 1 Timothy 4:8: "For bodily exercise profiteth little: but godliness is profitable unto all things, having promise of the life that now is, and of that which is to come."

At first glance, one might think that in this text Paul is scorning physical exercise. A closer study, however, reveals that he is simply comparing the importance of physical exercise to that of spiritual. Naturally, spiritual gains are more important than physical, though in some cases they are closely related. For example, a deepening commitment to Christ makes personal discipline a greater part of daily life. This in turn, carries over to controlled eating and activity, resulting in desired weight control.

Physical exercise is not to be compared with such things as Bible study and prayer, but it is important to good health and extremely valuable when trying to lose weight. Activity uses up calories. It's as simple as that!

The Combination That Works

Logic then brings us to a conclusion: We can control weight best by a combination of diet and exercise. If we neglect either, our efforts to control weight are likely to fail.

In one study, doctors observed 300 obese people who had each lost seventy pounds and kept it off. Of all the activities that these people performed daily, only two were held in common by all 300. They had *all* increased their physical activity and reduced the amount of fat they were eating.[1]

In another study, test groups were established to observe three different approaches to weight loss: diet alone, exercise alone, and a combination of diet and exercise. Each member of the diet group lost seven pounds; participants in the exercise group lost six pounds; and each of the combined diet and exercise group members lost thirteen pounds. More important, at both eight-week and twenty-four-week follow-ups, the combined diet and exercise group continued to lose weight, while the other groups did not.[2]

Exercise also makes a difference in the kind of weight we lose. Three groups of overweight women were put on a program designed to achieve a deficit of 500 calories per day. The diet only group decreased intake by 500 calories per day with no change in exercise. The exercise only group burned 500 calories per day with no change in caloric intake. The exercise and diet group ate 250 fewer calories per day and burned 250 calories by exercising. All three groups lost ten to twelve pounds; however, both the exercise only and the exercise and diet groups had greater reductions in body fat than the diet only group. The diet group actually experienced an undesirable loss in lean body weight.[3]

So, the best way to lose weight is obviously through a combination of reduced calories and increased activity. But this will demand a significant change in lifestyle for most of us. Americans have become some of the most inactive people in the world.

Inactivity: A Way of Life!

An executive sits at his desk during most of his working hours. A student sits in a classroom all day and in a library or in front of a television set at night.

Salespeople kill hours between customers, sitting at their desks or spending much of their day in automobiles traveling to various business appointments. Gadgets and appliances help us gain weight by opening our garage doors, washing our dishes, and even assisting the steering and braking of our cars.

A few years ago, our town was hit with a severe ice storm that began on New Year's Eve. Our electric power went out the next morning at 5:20 and interestingly did not return until 5:20 six days later. We didn't even have to reset our clocks.

During those six days I was impressed with the amount of labor involved in just existing. Water had to be carried in from an area that had electric power. We heated our house (or attempted to) with our fireplace. We had almost no wood on hand when the power went off, so we had to haul wood daily from ten miles away to keep the fire burning. Food had to be purchased from one of the few restaurants that was operating.

When the power returned, everything became easy again. Within a few minutes the house was warm, and water was ready at the tap. All the conveniences upon which we had depended daily were again available to serve us. But I'm not sure I will ever take them for granted. Being without them wasn't just inconvenient, it was hard work.

As a boy, I lived on a farm with no electric power. An ice storm like we experienced a few years ago would not have affected us on the farm because we were not dependent on outside energy to survive.

My mother's washer was made of wood and the tub had to be turned by hand to agitate the clothes. Fuel for keeping warm in winter was cut by hand—a yearly family project. Farm work was done with horses, and of course these had to be fed and cared for through the winter months, along with other livestock that helped provide our living. All of this effort expended calories.

Just think how things have changed.

The homemaker who used to spend 250 calories per hour doing her housework now has to burn only 120 calories because of her convenience appliances. Meanwhile, unless she finds ways to exercise, her savings account of calories is increasing, slowly but continually adding weight every day. Consider the wonders of this age that pamper us all, making us soft and overweight. I wonder how many pounds have been added to our frames as a result of installing automatic door openers in public buildings.

Fat is sneaky. It slips up on us.

A typist using a manual typewriter burns about 88 calories each hour. If she uses an electric typewriter, she will cut her calorie need to 73 hourly. At the end of the first week with her new typewriter, she will have stored 450 calories that would have been used up when she used a manual typewriter. If she doesn't cut her intake of food or increase her exercise, she will gain an extra pound every two months. At this rate, she will add thirty pounds in five years.

If you are serious about losing weight, you must fight fire with fire. You must begin looking for opportunities to exercise. And they are all around us.

Seize Opportunities for Exercise

For many years, I have jogged from parking spots to appointments. This not only helps me keep in shape but increases my efficiency because I make better use of my time. Seeing a man with a Bible under his arm run across a hospital parking lot toward the hospital may be startling to onlookers, causing them to conclude that someone is dying. How wrong they are! Someone is living!

You may need to eliminate an extension phone. The telephone company boasts that one extension phone saves the average person 76 miles of walking in a year. That saving of activity will add approximately two pounds in weight that you don't need. That's twenty pounds every ten years! When it comes to extra phones, you're better off to forget them and stick with the long distance, calorie-burning sprint to answer your single phone.

Since our children are all grown, we have thought for a number of years about getting a smaller home. One roadblock to that move has been the thought of living in a home without stairs. Stair climbing expends ten calories a minute. Think of the opportunities you have lost by calling up to your children instead of climbing the stairs to deliver a message. Also, remember the many times you have tossed dirty clothes down the basement stairs and missed the calorie-burning advantage of taking them down and walking up the stairs again.

Stop looking for the parking place nearest to your destination. You'll probably save time when you eliminate going around the block a half dozen times seeking a place to park, and the longer walk will fit into your daily exercise program.

Pass up elevators and escalators whenever possible. That is, of course, if your general health allows it (a rule that should apply to any exercise experience).

Go for a walk with your wife or husband. Your marriage may need the romance, and your body probably needs the exercise.

Walking is largely neglected in our mobile society. Yet it is an extremely healthful exercise, and a natural tranquilizer.

The American Medical Association says that a walk of just an extra mile each day for thirty-six days provides a pleasant way of shedding an extra pound. The extra mile is defined as just that—a mile of walking in addition to the amount you have been doing. So, by going the second mile, you can lose ten pounds a year, providing that you do not increase your calorie intake as you increase your exercise.

In their book, *Fitness Walking for Women*, authors Anne Kashiwa and James Rippe, M.D., point out four major contributions walking makes to a weight-loss program: it increases caloric expenditure, controls appetite, helps maintain resting metabolic rate, and burns fat while building muscle mass. (Resting metabolic rate is the term used for the amount of energy your body burns during rest.) So, regular walking may keep the caloric fires burning even when you have finished your healthful walk.[4]

According to Kashiwa and Rippe, walking is particularly good if you are extremely overweight, because higher impact activities such as running may be too hard on bones and joints.[5]

Pauline and I never tire of taking walks. When the weather permits, we like to walk about two miles daily. We walk along a scenic lake and up the highest hill in our county. As we break over the crest of Waterford Hill, we always thrill at the changes in beauty each season brings. Squirrels greet us along the way, as do neighborhood dogs.

One family started attending our church because of our walks. Seeing us walk by their house so many times caused them to become interested in our walk with the Lord and the ministry of our church which was located near their home. So we are confirmed believers in the value of walking.

Noting that pounds were melting off an overweight friend, I was prompted to ask him what he was doing to lose weight.

"I'm walking," he replied.

What a pleasant answer!

His method of becoming thin and trim was nothing mysterious: he was just walking.

Most people have time to walk.

Those who think they do not have time to enjoy walking could probably find the time by cutting down on television viewing. The average family spends between fifty and sixty hours weekly watching television, a pastime that uses few calories. Our two-mile walk takes less than one hour.

Sports are also good exercise. Team sports are fine when children are of school age, but as children grow into adults, they probably will not continue to participate in team sports. More enduring activities such as tennis and swimming can be shared by the whole family at all ages.

Bicycling is another excellent energy user that the entire family can enjoy. You are especially fortunate if you live in an area where paved bike trails are available. (Whether biking or walking, of course you must be mindful of safety.)

Cross-country skiing is another great exercise. When I first heard of this sport, I had little interest in it. Heading out across a field did not seem challenging to me; it sounded a bit boring. At Pauline's urging though, we tried cross-country skiing, and I enjoyed it so much that it is now one of my favorite activities.

You do not need special equipment for every form of exercise, but a few items can be very helpful. Exercise equipment doesn't have to be expensive. We have an exercise bike and a rowing machine, in addition to a few hand-held helps, such as, hand grips and weights to hold while doing other exercises. In the long run, these pieces of equipment cost far less than memberships in exercise clubs, and they are accessible at any time.

Below is a list of daily responsibilities and recreational activities, showing the calories used per hour. How many of these are a part of your life?

Activity	Approximate calories used per hour for:	
	130 lb. person	175 lb. person
Making a bed	247	332
Bicycling (fast)	520	700

	130 lb. person	175 lb. person
Calisthenics	247	332
Driving a car	117	157
Dishwashing	117	157
Eating	91	122
Football	468	630
Gardening	299	402
Golf	156	210
Ironing	130	175
Mopping floors	130	175
Office work	104	140
Painting (household)	156	210
Ping-Pong	325	427
Resting	65	88
Rowing	650	875
Sewing (machine)	91	122
Singing	117	157
Sweeping (broom)	143	192
Swimming	533	717
Tennis	364	490
Vacuuming	286	385
Walking fast	260	385
Writing	91	122
Running	481	647

We should be alert to opportunities for any extra motion or action that uses calories. Rather than pouting about having to do something extra, the Christian should cheerfully accept an active lifestyle. Imagine the changes this could bring to your life and home.

Redeeming the Time

Now, of course, Christians have far more at stake in life than losing weight. Each of us has been commissioned by our Lord to represent Him daily and to be part of His program of world evangelism. Since we want to represent our Lord well, this thought should add fervency to all we do. Paul wrote: "And whatsoever ye do, do it heartily, as to the Lord, and not unto men" (Col. 3:23).

As believers, we have responsibilities and work to do. And time is running out on us. I want to seize every opportunity to do things while I have time, and I want to do them fervently, as to the Lord.

What we do is important. *How* we do it may be even more important.

Jesus was the greatest example of one who gave Himself completely to every task. Wherever He went, the mundane was made miraculous. Everyday contacts were recognized as divine appointments. Common sights became teaching tools: the sower, the fig tree, the vine, and the branches. He made the most of every moment, living and dying with all His heart (Luke 23:32-43).

With Christ as their example, it is not surprising to find the New Testament writers calling for fervency in the Christian life. Paul urged the Christians in Rome to be fervent in spirit: "Not slothful in business; fervent in spirit; serving the Lord" (Rom. 12:11).

Peter asked his readers to be fervent in their love for one another: "Seeing ye have purified your souls in obeying the truth through the Spirit unto unfeigned love of the brethren, see that ye love one another with a pure heart fervently" (1 Peter 1:22).

James urged fervency in prayer: "The effectual fervent prayer of a righteous man availeth much" (James 5:16).

And those early Christians were fervent people! The word was out that they had "turned the world upside down" (Acts 17:6). We have the Gospel today because they gave themselves so fully to their task.

There are strong biblical grounds for getting on the move and living intensely. The message is vital, the time is short, and the need is great. The task is almost overwhelming. In light of this, we should give ourselves to every task energetically so that we will have additional opportunities to carry the message of Christ to others.

Bible heroes were men and women of action.

Consider Moses facing Pharaoh, producing plagues, dividing the sea, and leading that great multitude through the wilderness. And all this after he was eighty years old. Some senior citizen!

Paul pictured himself as an athlete. Outwardly, he didn't fit that image. But he seized each day for his Saviour and called upon his hearers to make the best use of every moment: "Redeeming the time," he called it (Eph. 5:16). He must have practiced what he preached for no one could have coasted through life and equaled Paul's accomplishments.

What was the dynamic that drove Paul on?

Let him tell it: "I press toward the mark for the prize of the high calling of God in Christ Jesus" (Phil. 3:14).

The Bible, then, calls for an active and intense life; it condemns idleness.

What does this have to do with losing weight?

Potentially a great deal.

We have learned that increased activity uses more energy and helps remove unwanted pounds. So get that mountain moving.

Rise earlier.

Attempt more.

Squeeze the life out of every second.

Learn to enjoy all the action of life whether it is work or play.

Enjoy All the Action of Life

I visited a young man in a hospital who had become paralyzed from his neck down as a result of an accident. It was his birthday, and he was having a good day in spite of his physical condition.

"God has given me a wonderful birthday present," he said.

"What's that?" I asked.

"I can move my thumb," he replied and demonstrated his new accomplishment for me. It was only a slight movement, but it was all he needed to brighten his day.

As I left that hospital room, I made my way down the corridor, opening and closing my hands and swinging my arms with a thankful heart. I had taken so much for granted. This injured man was grateful for so little.

Make the most of your ability to move by looking for opportunities to work, play, and be involved in the action of living. This will make every day an adventure and an experience in triumphant living.

Has your child spilled milk on your clean kitchen floor? Force yourself to remember what a small incident this is compared to famines in Africa! Although your instant reaction may be anger, learn the supernatural response of giving thanks that there is milk to spill at your house. Clean the floor with joy, seeing the episode as another opportunity for exercise.

Has someone neglected to do his job, leaving all the work to you? Ask God to help you be grateful for your privilege to be more productive and to make more calorie-consuming movements that will bring you another step closer to your weight loss goal.

Is the car dirty? Wash it with gusto.

Is the garage cluttered? Put it in order and praise God for a garage to clean. Thousands of people would like to have a place to live as spacious as your garage.

Stop being a spectator in your church.

Volunteer to teach a Sunday School class.

Join the choir.

Get involved in the church visitation program.

Take the responsibility of contacting those who have been absent from your church services.

Start a prayer group.

Distribute tracts to homes in your neighborhood.

Ask your pastor for some task that no one else wants to do and give it your best.

Follow Solomon's advice for fervent living: "Whatsoever thy hand findeth to do, do it with thy might" (Ecc. 9:10).

Your new lifestyle will make you a more effective servant of your Lord. You will also get a fat fringe benefit from your intense and active living: you'll be on your way to becoming thin, trim, and triumphant.

Questions for Application

1. Evaluate your current lifestyle. Are you actively involved in life, or are you more of a spectator?

2. What mechanical convenience could you live without in order to burn calories?

3. What type of physical exercise will you do this week? How often?

4. As a Christian, why should you be concerned about exercise?

8

The Fruit That Makes You Thin

A young woman who longed to be thin had her jaws wired together so she could eat no solid food. The wires remained until she had achieved her desired weight. Her method seems to have worked, but who wants to endure oral surgery every time pounds become a problem?

Three people I know have had their stomachs surgically stapled, cutting their capacity to take in food so that they could lose weight. One of these people died, another nearly died, and the third has had continuing health problems. The two who survived have taken off weight, but the price in pain and suffering has been high, to say nothing of the financial outlay invested in this method of becoming thin and trim.

A university professor, teaching a class in self-management skills, taught students who wanted to lose weight to give up some meaningful behavior every time they ate more calories than allowed in their diets. This could be as simple as giving up a favorite television program for a week or two.

Another approach the professor suggested was for the students to imagine themselves at their own funerals or bedridden with strokes as a result of overeating.

Should Christians resort to such immature imaginings or surgical manipulations?

Certainly not. There must be a better way.

A Better Way to Lose

The better way is within us in the person of the Holy Spirit. Since the Christian's body is His temple, this Divine Resident provides resources to keep His house in good condition. But if we are to receive the full advantage of these resources in daily life, we must surrender completely to Him.

Mendelssohn, the famous composer and musician, once visited a cathedral containing one of the most expensive organs in Europe. He listened to the organist practice and then asked permission to play.

"I don't know you," the organist replied, "and we don't allow strangers to play this organ."

At last the great musician persuaded the organist to let him play the expensive organ. As Mendelssohn played, the cathedral was filled with music more beautiful than the organist had ever heard. With tears in his eyes, he laid his hand upon Mendelssohn's shoulder and asked, "Who are you?"

"Mendelssohn," came the reply.

The organist was dumbfounded and embarrassed. "To think that an old fool like me nearly forbade Mendelssohn to play upon my organ!" he said.[1]

If we only knew what wonderful harmonies the Holy Spirit longs to bring to our lives, we would not rest until we had given Him full control.

But just what will happen if we surrender completely to the Holy Spirit? How will He change us? What will characterize our lives?

The Fruit of the Spirit

The purpose of the Holy Spirit is to reproduce the life of Jesus in us. And the Bible reveals what to expect when that happens: "But the fruit of the Spirit is love, joy, peace, long-suffering, gentleness, goodness, faith, meekness, temperance" (Gal. 5:22-23).

See how the Holy Spirit's control sets us free. Love is freedom from hate. Joy is freedom from depression. Peace is freedom from anxiety. Long-suffering is freedom from irritability. Gentleness is freedom from temper. Goodness is freedom from sin. Faith is freedom from doubt. Meekness is freedom from pride. Temperance is freedom from uncontrolled appetites; it is self-control.

Self-control is different from willpower because it is produced by the Holy Spirit working through us and is therefore adequate for every situation. Willpower is limited to human potential and often fails in a time of temptation or testing.

A dietician who learned that the title of one of my classes on weight loss was *The Fruit That Makes You Thin* seemed alarmed at what I might be teaching and asked what kind of fruit that could be.

"It is the fruit of the Spirit, which includes self-control," I explained.

"That makes sense to me," she said, obviously relieved.

Now we know how Paul could say he continually kept his body under control, bringing it into subjection so that he could run well in the race of life (1 Cor. 9:27). Since he was filled with the Holy Spirit, self-control was an inevitable result.

This is not new truth. We have all heard the dynamic testimonies of those with Spirit given self-control who have overcome alcohol or tobacco or drug addictions, fits of temper, and other recognized sins. But we have somehow ignored our need to overcome the sin of overeating. Reverend Pauley was one who recognized his intemperance in eating and lost 179 pounds. He explains:

> I confessed to the Lord that it was just as much a sin for me to overeat as to smoke or drink. It was the beginning of victory for me when I called it a sin. I could have called it a shortcoming, but it was a real sin and it was wrong.

Then I claimed the victory that God had given to alcoholics and nicotine addicts. I did what I had asked teens to do several times—put God to the test. I said that either He was the God who can give me the victory over this sin or He was not the God I thought He was, about whom I had preached through the years.

At that very moment, God gave me the victory.[2]

So, the same power was available to both Paul and Rev. Pauley, even though their experiences were separated by nearly 2,000 years. It must also be available to you and me.

"All right," you say. "I'm convinced. I believe the Holy Spirit produces self-control in believers. Why then do I not have enough discipline to control what I eat and how much I exercise?"

If you do not have self-control, the Holy Spirit is not in control of your life. You need to be filled with the Holy Spirit. The filling of the Holy Spirit is not an option for Christians but a matter of obedience: "And be not drunk with wine, wherein is excess; but be filled with the Spirit" (Eph. 5:18).

To be filled with the Spirit is to be controlled by the Spirit and therefore continually bring forth the fruit of the Spirit in daily living, including self-control.

But how can you be filled with the Holy Spirit?

You Must Stop Grieving the Spirit
If you long to be filled with the Holy Spirit, you must stop grieving Him.

And grieve not the Holy Spirit of God, whereby ye are sealed unto the day of redemption. Let all bitterness, and wrath, and anger, and clamor, and evil speaking, be put away from you, with all malice: And be ye kind one to another, tenderhearted, forgiving one another, even as God for Christ's sake hath forgiven you (Eph. 4:30-32).

Notice that these sins that grieve the Holy Spirit especially concern your attitude toward others.

You cannot be bitter toward others and be filled with the Holy Spirit. You cannot be angry with others and be filled with the Holy Spirit. You cannot gossip about others and be filled with the Holy Spirit. You cannot be filled with hatred and be filled with the Holy Spirit.

At the concluding service of a six-night series in an Alaskan church where I had been speaking, the pastor invited people to share what had happened in their lives that week. A woman stood and said, "The bitterness is gone."

What good words those are!

Repeat them if they are true in your life. If they are not true for you, confess to the Lord the sin of bitterness toward others and be rid of it.

Bitterness between believers is probably the greatest thief of power in churches and in the lives of Christians today.

Imagine bitterness, wrath, anger, clamor (angry shouting), and evil speaking being absent from your life, your home, your church. Now think of filling that void with kindness, tender-heartedness, forgiveness. This can become a reality for you simply by forgiving others as God for Christ's sake has forgiven you.

A woman who had been treated wrongly in her church shared her story with me. Though I was sympathetic to her wounds, I knew that her real problem was self-pity. The only source of deliverance from this sin would be a glimpse of her suffering Saviour.

"Has anyone spit upon you yet?" I asked.

"No," she replied, shocked by my question.

"They did on Jesus," I said. And suddenly she saw my point. While she had certainly been mistreated by people who should have known better, she had not endured nearly the suffering and pain Christ experienced in His death upon the cross for her sins.

My simple question changed her attitude about her persecutions, and she was able to forgive those who had snubbed and avoided her. As a result, she has become regular in the services of her church again and is unbothered by the backbiters and troublemakers.

Have you been grieving the Holy Spirit because of your bitterness, anger, and gossip? This might be the reason you have not been experiencing the fullness of the Spirit each day. Could your unwillingness to forgive be linked to your lack of self-control? Could your attitude toward others be keeping you from achieving your goal in weight control?

One morning our washer broke down in the middle of the week's washing, and I attempted to repair it. I replaced a switch and checked all the most likely reasons for a washer to quit. Nothing helped. Finally, I knelt beside the washer and prayed for guidance and then removed the back plate that covers the wiring one more time. There in plain sight was a wire hanging loose.

"I've found it!" I called upstairs to Pauline triumphantly. And within minutes the washer was working again.

One loose wire had broken the power connection.

Your negative relationships with others may be keeping you from experiencing the power of the Holy Spirit, manifested in self-control. Without this divine discipline as a part of your life, you will keep failing in your attempt to become thin and trim.

Your hate may determine your weight.

So, it is time to examine your life for things that grieve the Holy Spirit, especially your attitudes toward other people. As these wrong attitudes and actions are revealed to you, confess them immediately to your Lord. Then forsake and forget them: "If we confess our sins, He is faithful and just to forgive us our sins, and to cleanse us from all unrighteousness" (1 John 1:9). You cannot grieve the Holy Spirit and expect to experience His fruit in your life.

You Must Stop Quenching the Spirit

If you desire to be filled with the Spirit, you must also stop quenching the Holy Spirit: "Quench not the Spirit" (1 Thes. 5:19)

When we quench a fire, we stop it in its path. When we quench the Holy Spirit, we halt His work in us. We stifle or suppress Him. To quench the Holy Spirit is to resist Him, going our own way when His leading is clear.

To quench the Holy Spirit is to tune Him out when He speaks to us. All of us are familiar with tuning in and tuning out because radio and television have become such a part of our lives.

When our son, Tim, was very young, he went through a time of being troubled by nightmares, making it difficult for him to sleep through the night. We were concerned for him. Then, suddenly, he stopped talking about his nightmares and began sleeping without difficulty. When we asked about the change, he said, "When I get a bad dream, I just change channels."

Some of us change channels when the Holy Spirit speaks to us about what He wants to do in our lives. These channels may not be bad channels, just different channels which are full of thought patterns that center on anything other than what the Holy Spirit is speaking about at the moment.

Before we can recognize when we quench the Spirit, we need to know what the Holy Spirit desires to do in us.

We know that the Holy Spirit desires to comfort us. Jesus called the Holy Spirit the comforter, saying:

> And I will pray the Father, and He shall give you another Comforter, that He may abide with you for ever; even the Spirit of truth; whom the world cannot receive, because it seeth Him not, neither knoweth Him: but ye know Him; for He dwelleth with you, and shall be in you (John 14:16-17).

When we are in a state of fear, anxiety, or depression, we are unable to exercise proper self-control because our minds are occupied with problems that seem insurmountable. In these times, the Holy Spirit works to comfort us, taking away the fears and assuring us of God's love and care. He often

directs us to some Bible text to build our faith and put away
negativism. This faith builder will be just what we need to
remind us that temporary setbacks need not keep us from
reaching our goals in weight control.

But if we quench Him in His efforts to comfort us, we will
lack His filling or control. Receiving His comfort will allow us
to relax in our Lord's care and will cause the fruit of the Spirit
to grow in us.

The comforting work of the Holy Spirit may also be
intended to relieve us of guilt. Overweight people are often
tormented with guilt because of failing to lose weight when
they have attempted to do so. They may also be oppressed by
guilt over some sin in the past that has been confessed and
forgiven but that still drags them down into depression. The
Holy Spirit works to take away that guilt by reminding those
under such self-condemnation that sins confessed are sins forgiven. To reject this good news is to quench the Holy Spirit
and thereby forbid His fruit to grow in our lives.

The Holy Spirit also desires to teach us: "But the Comforter,
which is the Holy Ghost, whom the Father will send in My
name, He shall teach you all things, and bring all things to
your remembrance, whatsoever I have said unto you" (John
14:26).

We have so much to learn. All the experiences of life have
lessons to teach us. The goal of the Holy Spirit's teaching is to
make us more like Jesus. He longs to show us God's love in
every trial and triumph so that we will develop into Christlike
people. That is the message of Romans 8:28-29:

> And we know that all things work together for good to
> them that love God, to them who are the called ac-
> cording to His purpose. For whom He did foreknow,
> He also did predestinate to be conformed to the image
> of His Son, that He might be the firstborn among many
> brethren.

When we rebel at experiences that come to us, we are

quenching the Holy Spirit and thereby resisting His control. The Holy Spirit desires to guide us into all truth:

> Howbeit when He, the Spirit of truth, is come, He will guide you into all truth: for He shall not speak of Himself; but whatsoever He shall hear, that shall He speak: and He will show you things to come. He shall glorify Me: for He shall receive of Mine, and shall show it unto you (John 16:13-14).

The Bible is the source of truth, and every word has been given by inspiration through the Holy Spirit. He longs to reveal the deep truths and mysteries of Scripture to us, but this requires us to take the time to study the Bible and listen to those whom God has given to the church as teachers. As we study, faith grows, and we learn more about our Lord. This enriching time in Bible study glorifies Jesus and equips us to tell others about Him.

To neglect personal devotional study and the services of the church is to quench the Holy Spirit. When we do this, we are weakened spiritually and are likely to be defeated in any area of effort at the time, including that of shedding those extra pounds.

The Holy Spirit desires to empower us as witnesses to the world of Christ's love, His sacrifice on the cross, and His resurrection. This message has been entrusted to us to share with the world. We are to be witnesses of the Gospel to all we meet and to people everywhere.

> But ye shall receive power, after that the Holy Ghost is come upon you: and ye shall be witnesses unto Me both in Jerusalem, and in all Judea, and in Samaria, and unto the uttermost part of the earth (Acts 1:8).
>
> And when they had prayed, the place was shaken where they were assembled together; and they were all filled with the Holy Ghost, and they spoke the word of God with boldness (Acts 4:31).

What part do you play in world evangelism? In reaching your community? In witnessing to those with whom you work or come in contact socially?

Have you been quenching the Holy Spirit when He has opened opportunities to share the Gospel with others? Are you missing out on the thrilling, active life of one who is involved in community and world evangelism? If so, you will ultimately feel this loss in every part of life: spiritual, emotional, and physical.

In short, the Holy Spirit has a ministry in every area of your life. When you yield to Him, you are in tune with the purpose of God for you. When you tune Him out, you are quenching Him.

When you stop quenching the Holy Spirit and yield to Him day by day, some wonderful things will begin to happen.

Your day will unfold as a part of His plan.

You will notice opportunities that you would have missed before.

You will begin to sense the timing of the Lord in all things because you are being led by the Holy Spirit and becoming sensitive to His direction.

You will be more aware of temptation and more able to overcome it in His power. Your appetite will be tempered by His leading and wisdom. Whatever you eat or drink will be done to the glory of God.

The Lord's calming voice will comfort you when everything seems to be falling apart. Life's irritations will be recognized as experiences that give opportunity for you to be patient and long-suffering.

The needs of others will be brought to your attention and you will be refreshed in ministering to them. Having your own way will become less important. Allowing the Holy Spirit to have His way in your life will receive priority. And as the Holy Spirit is allowed to direct your life daily, the fruit of the Spirit will be evident in you, including self-control, so important in winning the weight war.

You will find yourself responding to Bible instruction that

you learned long ago but had been ignoring.

Others will notice that you have an attitude of thanksgiving and praise, even on difficult days.

You will be constantly conscious of the presence of the Lord, which will keep you sensitive to His leading.

One evening as I was returning home from hospital visitation, I felt impressed to go to the home of a young family that had just begun attending our church. It was nearly time for our evening meal, but the name of this family kept coming to mind, so I turned my car around and headed back to the city where they lived.

When I arrived at the door of this home, the wife answered my knock in tears. Her husband was in another room with a gun, intending to take his life.

I made my way cautiously into the room where he was sitting with a shotgun across his knees and sat down beside him.

After reading a portion of the Bible to him and praying for him, this troubled man laid the gun aside. He is still alive these many years later. I am so glad that I did not quench the Holy Spirit that day as He led me to a home where I could be instrumental in saving a man's life.

As we yield to the Holy Spirit daily and stop quenching Him in His work in our lives, the fruit of the Spirit will keep on being produced in us.

So, stop tuning out the Holy Spirit. You cannot quench the Holy Spirit and expect to experience His fruit in your life. The moment you try to go it alone, self-control will disappear. You will be back on that old treadmill called "willpower" and from there it is but a short distance to gimmicks and failure again.

You Must Walk in the Spirit

Finally, if you long to be filled with the Holy Spirit, you must walk in the Spirit: "This I say then, walk in the Spirit, and ye shall not fulfill the lust of the flesh" (Gal. 5:16).

Walking demonstrates faith.

Jesus told the man who had been sick of the palsy that he

was to take up his bed and walk. That demanded faith. He had not been able to walk. The fact that he arose and walked at the Lord's command gave evidence of his confidence in the power of Christ (Matt. 9:2-7).

Peter walked on the water to go to Jesus. That was a walk of faith. When Peter's faith faltered, he began to sink (Matt. 14:28-31). It was faith that made that miraculous walk on the sea possible.

The person who walks in the Spirit has taken the filling of the Holy Spirit by faith after having confessed his grieving and quenching of the Spirit in full surrender of heart.

Such a person demonstrates the fruit of the Spirit: love, joy, peace, long-suffering, gentleness, goodness, faith, meekness, and temperance (self-control).

Self-control. How we need it! The Bible paints a tragic picture of the person who lacks it: "He that hath no rule over his own spirit is like a city that is broken down and without walls" (Prov. 25:28).

Be Filled with the Spirit

Be Filled with the Spirit. That is your need. You will no longer be like a city that is broken down and without walls. Self-control will bring order to every part of your life, even to your effort to lose weight. The fruit of the Spirit is indeed the fruit that makes you thin.

One further word. The filling of the Spirit is *not a one-time experience.* Unlike the baptism of the Spirit, the filling of the Spirit is needed whenever we allow the old sin nature to assume control. You will not have to be told when that happens.

Thankfully, God's formula for filling is always at hand: confess your sins of grieving and quenching the Holy Spirit in full surrender of heart and will. The moment you give Him control of your life all will be well again. His power will be yours so that you can become all you ought to be—a triumphant believer whose life is under the control of our faithful and loving Lord.

Questions for Application

1. Think of someone you know who has surrendered to the Holy Spirit. What qualities do you most admire in this person?

2. What is keeping the Holy Spirit from controlling your life? Have you grieved or quenched the Spirit?

3. What action will you take to allow the Spirit to have full control of your life?

9

Discipline:
How Sweet It Is!

Recently, I visited a man whom I had not seen in several months and hardly recognized. At our last meeting, he had been overweight and out of shape. Now he had lost forty pounds and appeared athletic and healthy. He was clearly on a different course in life and was enjoying it.

A woman with whom I shared the dentist's waiting room had been addicted to tobacco. Her husband had urged her to quit smoking many times but to no avail. As we talked while awaiting our dental appointments, she told me of finally ending her bondage to nicotine. Her freedom was like a breath of fresh air, and she was glad to talk about it. "Stopping smoking was one of the easiest things I have ever done," she said. The power to stop smoking had been within her since the day she received Christ as her Saviour, but she had not used that power and so had been in bondage when freedom was well within her reach. The moment she yielded that area of her life to Christ, victory came with ease.

A man I met at the shopping mall told me of the change in his life since reading *Weight! A Better Way to Lose.* He had lost more than seventy pounds and was pleased with his new lifestyle.

These three victors have all experienced the delight of discipline; the exhilarating sense of freedom that comes from being able to refuse things that are not good for us and choose those that enrich our lives.

Discipline is the outworking of the inner work of the Holy Spirit called self-control. It is self-control in action.

Biblical Examples of Disciplined Living

Joseph knew the joy of a disciplined life and it paid off for him. Sold into slavery by his brothers, he remained steadfast in faith and character even in adversity. When Potiphar's wife tried to seduce him while her husband was away, Joseph refused her advances and as a result was falsely accused and placed in prison. Even there, he retained his faith and integrity and ultimately was exalted to one of the top positions in Egypt. His disciplined life finally brought the fulfillment of his dreams and reunited him with his family (Gen. 39–50).

Daniel became a captive in Babylon while still a young man. The temptation to go along with the idolatrous and loose living there must have been very strong. But Daniel chose a life of discipline and let his decision be made known soon after being taken into captivity. Selected to be one of King Nebuchadnezzar's advisers, he was offered special treatment if he would compromise his convictions, but he chose instead the joy of discipline:

> But Daniel purposed in his heart that he would not
> defile himself with the portion of the king's meat, nor
> with the wine which he drank: therefore he requested
> of the prince of the eunuchs that he might not defile
> himself (Dan. 1:8).

Because Daniel's self-discipline had to do with abstaining from certain kinds of food, those who long to lose weight today can identify with his need of inner strength to overcome the urge to eat from the king's menu. The tempting aroma of meat and rich pastries being cooked for the king and other members of his staff must have intensified the struggle that Daniel, Shadrach, Meschach, and Abednego endured while eating their daily portions of vegetables and drinking only water. But imagine their satisfaction after ten days on their chosen diet when they appeared healthier than those who had eaten at the king's table.

Daniel was also disciplined in his prayer life. When his enemies conspired to have him thrown into a den of hungry lions if he worshiped anything but the golden image the king had made, Daniel kept on worshiping God and making request of Him for his needs and desires. Knowing that the king had signed a decree that would carry out the desires of his enemies, this disciplined man of faith still continued praying three times a day as he had been doing before this life threatening situation had developed:

> Now when Daniel knew that the writing was signed,
> he went into his house; and his windows being open
> in his chamber toward Jerusalem, he kneeled upon his
> knees three times a day, and prayed, and gave thanks
> before his God, as he did aforetime (Dan. 6:10).

Was this discipline worthwhile?

Review the scene at the lions' den the morning after Daniel was thrown in to die and judge for yourself. King Darius regretted sentencing Daniel to die and spent the night fasting and unable to sleep. At the first light of day, he hurried to the lions' den to see whether or not Daniel had survived the night. Upon reaching the den, he called out to Daniel, asking if his God had been able to deliver him from the lions. Daniel answered that God had sent an angel to shut the mouths of the lions and that he had not been injured (Dan. 6:21-22).

Why not?

He knew how to pray effectively when the crisis came because he was disciplined in prayer.

The *Reader's Digest Great Encyclopedia Dictionary* defines discipline as: "Training of the mental, moral, and physical powers by instruction, control, and exercise."

Control and exercise are the key words in this study. The whole plan is built around them. But we have also learned that a believer's approach to achieving control is different and far more effective than that of an unbeliever.

While unbelievers may have some success at increasing discipline through building self-confidence or using other psychological techniques, believers can yield to the Holy Spirit and have discipline as a natural result of that surrender.

Exchanging Self-confidence for Faith

Earlier in my life I had great difficulty controlling my nerves when speaking or singing in public. Sometimes my voice would tremble, and often my knees felt shaky. Focusing on my training or natural ability fell far short of meeting my need.

Researchers say the number one fear among Americans is speaking before a crowd, and I could certainly identify with that anxiety.

I tried again and again to build up self-confidence enough to overcome those trembling times, but nothing seemed to help. Then I decided to exchange my self-confidence for Christ-confidence. By trading my self-confidence for faith, I was able to achieve the discipline I needed to sing or speak publically without fear. I stopped trying to convince myself that I was adequate for the occasion and started depending entirely on Christ (Gal. 3:3). Now I am at ease before large and small groups because I draw my discipline from the Lord.

Discipline is absolutely necessary in the life of anyone desiring to become thin and trim, but let us understand that our need goes beyond just determination. We are talking about divine discipline that is available to every Christian because the Holy Spirit is within us. Peter called this being partakers of the divine nature (2 Peter 1:4).

An alcoholic who was being urged to "hold on to sobriety" said, "I need someone to hold me." The love of God makes that kind of security possible. As we rest full faith in Christ, He holds us and His strength becomes ours. That is why Paul could say, "I can do all things through Christ which strengtheneth me" (Phil. 4:13). What a good faith builder to place on the refrigerator door!

Exchanging Willpower for God's Power

How do you intend to desert those high calorie finales at the next big dinner you attend?

With willpower?

You may pull it off this time, but your determination isn't likely to last.

Has willpower been sufficient for you to win over temptation in the past?

Probably not.

And that is the reason you are reading this book. You are looking for a way to win and *keep* on winning . . . and losing.

Part of your solution will be to understand the weakness of your own willpower. All human willpower is limited, and the sooner you realize this the better.

Peter was convinced that he had willpower enough to keep from denying his Lord under any circumstances. "Though all men shall be offended because of Thee, yet will I never be offended," he declared (Matt. 26:33).

Jesus replied, "Verily I say unto thee, That this night, before the cock crow, thou shalt deny Me thrice" (Matt. 26:34).

Still confident, Peter said, "Though I should die with Thee, yet will I not deny Thee" (Matt. 26:35).

You know the rest of the story.

Before long, Peter was denying his Lord and cursing and swearing (Matt. 26:69-75). The breakdown of his willpower brought guilt, tears, and regret:

> And after a while came unto him they that stood by, and said to Peter, Surely thou also art one of them; for thy speech betrayeth thee. Then began he to curse and to swear, saying, I know not the man. And imme-

diately the cock crew. And Peter remembered the word of Jesus, which said unto him, Before the cock crow, thou shalt deny Me thrice. And he went out, and wept bitterly (Matt. 26:73-75).

Poor Peter.

He had thought his willpower would be enough to handle the situation and it was not. No wonder he later wrote about believers being partakers of the divine nature, kept by the power of God. At last he had learned that he was in need of power beyond his own to overcome temptation.

Thankfully, that unlimited power is available to us. Though our strength may be small, we are invited to trade our weakness for His strength:

> He giveth power to the faint; and to them that have no might He increaseth strength. Even the youths shall faint and be weary, and the young men shall utterly fall: But they that wait upon the Lord shall renew their strength; they shall mount up with wings as eagles; they shall run, and not be weary; and they shall walk, and not faint (Isa. 40:29-31).

Discipline in Eating

Becky Kirkman learned about the delight of discipline at a Christian weight control class. The teacher challenged the class to go without sugar for two weeks. It was then that Becky became aware of the hold sugar had on her. She says the first few days were really tough but in going without sugar for two weeks, she lost six pounds.

Becky has now discovered that she has a heart problem and is grateful to have already arrived at her goal in weight control. She writes:

> *I am grateful for the knowledge I have gained from your book in taking off my excess weight and learning to main-*

tain it. It may prevent a minor heart attack from becoming a major one. I am now at 123 pounds and feel great! I am so glad I didn't give up and let the weight keep creeping up five pounds at a time.

Becky has chosen a disciplined lifestyle and believes it is the way to live for the rest of her life. She says:

Through these classes I began to realize that diet isn't a one or two week commitment. It is for LIFE, and your life should belong to the Lord.

I agree. And not just because it makes weight control possible. The benefits of a disciplined life are so great that they are worth attaining whether or not weight is a factor.

When my doctor told me to avoid sugar, I realized this was going to bring about a major lifestyle change for me. Sweets had become a very important part of my life. I thoroughly enjoyed chocolate milkshakes, hot fudge sundaes, chocolate chip cookies, cheesecake, blueberry pie, and dozens of other delicious concoctions that are all loaded with sugar.

Now I refuse all such treats with ease.

Have I lost my taste or desire for them?

No.

Could I enjoy them again?

Certainly.

But I have found something sweeter: self-discipline. I experience a sweet satisfaction in knowing that I am no longer under the control of a substance called sugar. Discipline has brought a sense of freedom that I did not have before, which cannot be found in indulgence. I have been set free.

This is an important lesson to learn: Discipline sets us free! And this is true whether the issue is eating or refusing certain foods or controlling our moods and tempers.

You do not have to be in bondage to deserts or depression.

You do not have to be ruled by calories or a complaining attitude.

God has equipped you to live triumphantly:

> But thanks be to God, which giveth us the victory
> through our Lord Jesus Christ. Therefore, my beloved
> brethren, be ye steadfast, unmoveable, always abound-
> ing in the work of the Lord, forasmuch as ye know that
> your labor is not in vain in the Lord (1 Cor. 15:57-58).

Discipline and Positive Living

Discipline is also vital to positive living. Too often, we limit
our thinking about discipline to the things we should not be
doing. Discipline is equally important in moving us to do
things that we ought to be doing.

A number of people have asked me to read through book
manuscripts when they were finished, but only a few have
actually brought me manuscripts to read. The reason for this is
the amount of discipline required to write a book. Many believe they have worthy stories to tell, but few discipline themselves enough to put them in writing.

Discipline moves us forward.

You will be interrupted many times in your devotional time,
and you will be tempted to become discouraged and stop
your daily Bible study and prayer. Nevertheless, these important faith builders are well worth the demands you must make
on yourself to keep on with them.

Taking steps toward becoming thin and trim will require
discipline, especially in seeking activity. You are sure to find it
easier to put off taking daily walks or doing calisthenics than to
discipline yourself to carry through on this important part of
your new lifestyle.

Your favorite chair will beckon.

The television set will call.

But you must shut out these distractions until after you have
been sufficiently active to stay on track with your weight control goals. Every time you give in to the temptation to choose
ease instead of action, you add to your problem. Of course
you will need times of rest and recreation, but discipline will

be required to keep a properly balanced lifestyle.

With the passing of years, I have become extremely conscious of the value of time and the importance of investing it wisely. I rise earlier now because this gives me more time for action than I would have by oversleeping. The countdown of life continues relentlessly for all of us. If we are to become what we want to be and accomplish as much as possible, we must be disciplined about what we do and how we use the time that remains.

Discipline for the Sake of Others

Our personal discipline also affects others. If we are out of control and up and down in our relationship to God, others will be adversely affected. Our witness for Christ will be weak and inconsistent. On the other hand, discipline of our lives can make us effective witnesses for our Lord.

This was Paul's concern when he faced the question of whether or not to eat meat that had been offered to idols. He knew that the idols were nothing (1 Cor. 8:4), but he was concerned about the tender consciences of those who did not know this and therefore might be offended by his eating of this meat. As a result, he urged his readers in Corinth to be careful lest their liberty in Christ cause them to be stumbling blocks to others. He concludes: "Wherefore, if meat make my brother to offend, I will eat no flesh while the world standeth, lest I make my brother to offend" (1 Cor. 8:13)

I am constantly aware that I must be careful about what I eat because others expect me to be an example of self-discipline. Some who watch and follow me have hypoglycemia, and others need to lose weight. Recently, at a banquet where I was the speaker, a man said he would be watching to see what I chose to eat and would be doing the same. Since my lifestyle has been established for many years, I could have broadened my choices a bit without dire consequences, but then I would have failed my friend. Discipline in eating that night was especially satisfying because I knew by keeping within the bounds of my diet, I was imparting strength to another.

Generally, people lose weight more easily when they meet as a class or a fellowship because they can help each other conquer the problem. Discipline becomes easier when others share the load and encourage one another. Building one another up through personal discipline makes any sacrifice worthwhile and the whole experience more satisfying.

Remembering your responsibility to others will probably make a difference the next time you eat out with friends. Instead of cheating on your diet and laughing it off as human frailty, you will be conscious of how your discipline affects others. Contributing to the failure of another who longs to be thin and trim is no laughing matter.

Taking the long look, self-discipline is one way of laying up treasures in heaven. The Bible contains many promises of rewards for overcomers. These rewards have to do in part with overcoming temptation. And that's what personal discipline is all about.

Do not think of discipline as something that makes life drab and boring. On the contrary, it is what adds challenge and adventure to life. All believers are in a constant battle with the world, the flesh, and the devil. Discipline is the outward evidence of victory.

Conduct yourself like a conquering general at the supermarket, at the dinner table, and at snack time. Meet the challenge of high calorie eating and overcome it. Engage laziness and disorderly living and win.

Enjoy the disciplined life.

It is the only life that gives constant evidence of the presence of the indwelling Holy Spirit.

It is the only life that satisfies and ministers to others.

Discipline assures ultimate success while giving a present sense of accomplishment.

How sweet it is!

Questions for Application

1. What are the weaknesses of human willpower?

2. In what specific areas do you need to become more disciplined? How can you accomplish this?

3. How does your discipline, or lack of discipline, affect those you love?

10

Shape Up Your Marriage

Married losers have a lot to gain, like improved health, fewer emotional hang-ups, and a longer life together.

These are gains worth achieving.

Marriage is under fire today. The pressures of our fast-paced way of life and the dropping of old moral standards have taken a deadly toll on many marriages that started well. My counseling work and that of friends who specialize in marriage counseling show that even Christian homes are feeling the strain of the age, and many of them are breaking up. One practical step to take in strengthening our marriages is to keep our weight under control so that we will be healthy and attractive.

Christian married couples have a lot going for them that should enable them to stand through the storms and endure. Bible reading and prayer in the home ought to be a daily spiritual discipline that strengthens the marriage bond. Involvement in the work of Christ through the local church ought to add inspiration and purpose to life. The ministry of the Bible in public worship services ought to aid in building a home on a solid foundation. But these activities alone cannot guarantee a good marriage.

Good health and emotional well-being are also important factors in a meaningful marriage. Since it has already been shown that being overweight affects both of these areas of life, it makes sense to know what to do when fat invades the family.

Perhaps you are not sure whether weight is a problem in your marriage.

■ Can you still wear your wedding gown?

■ Is your suit or tuxedo size the same as it was on your wedding day?

■ Do you fit as comfortably in each other's arms now as you did then?

■ Does your wedding ring still fit?

■ Are you concerned about weight causing your mate to wander?

■ Has your husband told you that he now has more wife to love?

■ Has your wife mentioned a "spare tire" when automobiles are not the topic of conversation?

■ Has she inquired about the status of your life insurance?

■ Would (could) he still carry you over the threshold?

■ Did you get a Weight-Watcher's membership for Christmas?

If you'd rather not answer any of the above questions, it is time to get serious about weight control

The Closest Bond on Earth

Married people who are trying to lose weight have an advantage over singles because their close bond makes it possible to help one another in unique ways. This is in keeping with God's purpose for marriage in the beginning: "The Lord God said, 'It is not good that the man should be alone: I will make him an help meet for him'" (Gen. 2:18).

How close is this bond?

Read Adam's answer to our question:

And Adam said, 'This is now bone of my bones, and

> flesh of my flesh: she shall be called woman, because she was taken out of man. Therefore shall a man leave his father and his mother, and shall cleave unto his wife: and they shall be one flesh (Gen. 2:23-24).

The marriage bond is strengthened when both husband and wife develop a close relationship with Christ. An important dimension to this commitment to Christ and each other is the bond of prayer. As husbands and wives pray for one another's needs, they draw closer together.

I have shared a description of Pauline's devotional and exercise time with thousands. Each morning she spends time alone reading her Bible, praying, and exercising. I know that she brings my needs before God in prayer daily and this deepens our relationship. No need that I have is too personal for her to know or to tell God in prayer. She also knows that I intercede for her each day, for both physical and spiritual needs.

Should a husband or wife be praying fervently for an overweight mate to win the battle of the bulge?

Absolutely.

Knowing that the loved one is involved in even this sensitive, personal desire makes the heavy spouse confident of success and strengthens the marriage relationship.

Husbands and wives can also fight the battle of the bulge by doing things together that use up calories. They can take walks at any hour of the day or night and improve their communication skills while they shed pounds. They can become involved in organized athletic activities or even do calisthenics together. Creative couples find many calorie-burning opportunities to share. How creative are you?

The husband or wife of the hopeful loser can become the key encourager of the one who is trying hard to become thin and trim.

How important this is!

There is no place in a marriage for sarcastic and cutting remarks about those we love when they become overweight. Thoughtless words, even words spoken in a joking manner, may inflict lasting wounds.

Sometimes when either the husband or wife gains a considerable amount of weight, barriers grow between them that hinder their relationship. This should not be true, but it happens.

"It's her weight," said a young husband who was trying to explain why he has lost interest in showing affection to his wife.

Similar comments may come from wives whose husbands have become careless about their weight. True love continues when pounds increase. And the wise mate will do his or her part in helping a loved one overcome the problem of being overweight.

Why Do Married People Gain Weight?

There are a number of reasons why people gain weight after the wedding day, but one of the most obvious is a change in eating habits. These changes vary with individuals and couples, but if you're heavier now than on your wedding day, you've likely increased your intake of calories.

Maybe too much eating out is the cause of those added pounds that have become a part of you: too much pizza, too many big burgers and fries, too many sugar-packed soft drinks. In short, you may be the victim of a busy schedule that sends both you and your spouse to fast food restaurants too often.

Perhaps one of you is a gourmet cook, and having your own kitchen has given the fancied chef an opportunity to try some new creations that are loaded with calories. The meals have been delicious and different, but now you're both living proof of the cook's culinary talents, and you need to come up with a recipe for becoming thin and trim again.

Strange as it may seem, marital bliss can increase weight. Happiness can actually add to a weight problem if it leads to hearty eating together in celebration of shared joy. Eating out in fine restaurants with romantic settings and rich food can give both the husband and wife more partner to love.

Sometimes pounds are added by the stress of new responsibilities brought on by married life. Concern over unpaid bills, disobedient children, marital strife, and other pressures have sent many husbands and wives to the refrigerator in the night hours to snack and try to forget. The catch in this kind of diversion is that it only adds another problem, that of becoming overweight.

Pregnancies also produce pounds. With each child a woman may have added more weight than she lost after the birth. A letter that I received recently told of this happening to the writer. She wrote to tell me how her new lifestyle, based on *Weight! A Better Way to Lose,* had helped her regain her desired weight.

Some couples have a hard time pinpointing the reason for their increased weight. They were not aware of any fast gain but can hardly believe their eyes when looking at their wedding pictures. In some of these cases, advancing age may be partly to blame for weight gain. Fewer calories are required to maintain weight as we reach maturity. Yet, food intake is often unchanged. When this happens, the result, of course, is predictable.

Then there are those who were overweight when they were married.

"He knew I was fat when he married me!"

Does that mean you should go on punishing yourself and injuring your health after your wedding?

Think about it!

There's a better way to live.

Love and Emotional Well-Being

Overweight marrieds should consider taking off pounds by reawakening their love life.

After marriage, the responsibilities of life often rob couples of the freshness of new love. Both the husband and wife may begin to hurt emotionally and are likely to let down standards of eating and activity that have kept them healthy and attractive. A reawakening of love can provide emotional nourishment and make it possible to overcome this problem.

While in our first pastorate, we were entertaining an evangelist and his wife in our home while they were holding a week of meetings at our church. On Sunday morning, Pauline and I were ready for church a bit earlier than the other couple and were waiting for them. Seizing the opportunity, I took Pauline in my arms and kissed her. At that moment the evangelist walked into the room, taking us by surprise.

"The revival is on!" he shouted.

How many calories are burned up in a kiss?

I don't know. But I do know that a warm and loving relationship in a home makes success in any effort by either partner more likely. This kind of a revival in your marriage might give birth to the kind of lifestyle that brings everything into proper perspective, including the encouragement and activity needed to conquer family weight problems.

The two people sitting across the desk from me were not young lovers. They were approaching sixty, but had the same stars in their eyes that I have seen so many times in those much younger. These two had come to talk to me about becoming one. They were in love, and we were planning their wedding.

Turning to the prospective groom, I asked him about their honeymoon.

"It's going to be a long one," he replied.

And he had the right idea; the one I've been trying to get across to brides and grooms for more than thirty years.

Why should young newlyweds be the greatest lovers? Why shouldn't loving improve with age? The passing of years should mature affection, making it richer and more thrilling.

The lament of Jesus concerning the condition of the church at Ephesus, revealed in His letter to that church in the Book of Revelation, would be a fitting statement on the climate of love between too many husbands and wives: "Nevertheless I have somewhat against thee, because thou hast left thy first love" (Rev. 2:4).

Nothing is more tragic than declining love, whether it is true of a marriage relationship, the state of things within a local church, or our walk with Christ. In any of these situations, declining love speaks of cooling affection, of just going through the motions in a setting where things much warmer and better are to be expected.

What is the temperature of love in your marriage?

Has love declined?

Do you remember a better day?

Christian couples should remember that their love for each other is intended to be a picture of Christ's love for the church. This great mystery is revealed in Paul's letter to the Ephesian church and is described as follows:

> Husbands, love your wives, even as Christ also loved the church, and gave Himself for it; that He might sanctify and cleanse it with the washing of water by the word, that He might present it to Himself a glorious church, not having spot, or wrinkle, or any such thing; but that it should be holy and without blemish. So ought men to love their wives as their own bodies. He that loveth his wife loveth himself. For no man ever yet hated his own flesh; but nourisheth and cherisheth it, even as the Lord the church: For we are members of His body, of His flesh, and of His bones. For this cause shall a man leave his father and his mother, and shall be joined unto his wife, and they two shall be one flesh. This is a great mystery: but I speak concerning Christ and the church. Nevertheless let every one of you in particular so love his wife even as himself; and the wife see that she reverence her husband (Eph. 5:25-33).

There are, then, some parallels between the love of Christ for the church and the love of a man for his wife that contain valuable lessons for married people.

Sacrificial Love

The love of Christ for His church is a sacrificial love.

Love always causes us to give: "For God so loved the world,

that He gave His only begotten Son, that whosoever believeth in Him should not perish, but have everlasting life" (John 3:16).

You can give without loving, but you cannot love without giving.

A woman once told me that her marriage had been changed by something her pastor had said in one of his sermons.

Immediately interested, I asked what he had said that had made such a difference in her home.

She replied that he had said, "You may be asking whether or not you are getting enough out of your marriage, when that is not the right question. You should be asking whether or not your husband or wife is getting all that *he* or *she* should be getting out of the marriage."

The pastor's thought-provoking question had turned their marriage around and made them givers as well as receivers. And that's what love is all about.

You may want to become a giver by lovingly helping your mate change eating habits so that he or she will lose weight. This kind of giving will start before you go to the store, when you are planning your meals for the week.

In order to do this kind of planning, you will need to become aware of the calorie content of foods that are part of your lifestyle. You will especially want to guard against purchasing diet busters that pile up calories and put on pounds. Foods high in sugar are notorious for doing this. And many foods that find their way to our tables with regularity are loaded with sugar.

A twelve ounce soft drink contains approximately nine teaspoons of sugar.

In some presweetened breakfast cereals, more than half of what you get is sugar, nearly three teaspoons per ounce.

One of the best ways to cut down on calories is simply to stop buying and making high calorie foods. This is true of ending any addiction.

"I'd sure like to quit smoking," a defeated man said.

"Why do you carry cigarettes in your pocket?" I asked.

When temptation is within reach, we are likely to yield to it. So keep those diet destroyers out of reach. Stop buying them. Paul describes this route to victory as follows:

> Let us walk honestly, as in the day; not in rioting and drunkenness, not in chambering and wantonness, not in strife and envying. But put ye on the Lord Jesus Christ, and make not provision for the flesh, to fulfill the lusts thereof (Rom. 13:13-14).

How simple.

If you stop making provision for the weakness of the flesh, you will stop losing battles to the flesh.

Love will, of course, move wives and husbands to discuss the guidelines of eating and exercise before embarking on a new lifestyle that is drastically different for both of them. This will help keep peace in the family and foster a growing relationship where both can rejoice in their progress in weight control.

The husband and wife who start looking for ways to please each other will not be disappointed. This desire to give will change the whole mood of their marriage. Shaping up their relationship will help them consume their savings account of unneeded calories, speeding them on to their combined goal of becoming thin and trim.

Love That Is Expressed Often

Finally, the love of Christ is a love that is expressed often.

How long has it been since you expressed your love to your wife or husband? A day? A week? A month? A year? If it has been a long time since you have communicated your love in either word or act, you are not living as God intended (1 Cor. 7:1-5). Your lack of expressed love may be hindering your ability or your mate's ability to become all you both long to be.

Keep your love alive. Look for opportunities to show your love.

What do you like about your wife? Is she kind? Generous?
Talented? Godly? Industrious? These and other qualities she
may have are excellent reasons to walk across the room and
take her in your arms. Every positive point she possesses provides another excuse for showing your love to her. These acts
of love may involve doing things that get you more active,
such as, doing things she wants to do or going places she
wants to go. This extra action may help you to become thin
and trim. Expressing love may also mean taking more time
with your wife, sharing her feelings and encouraging her in
the effort she is making to become healthier and more desir-
able to you.

What is there about your husband that made you choose
him to be your man? Is he strong? Gentle? Faithful? God-
fearing? Hardworking? Make a list of his strengths and tell him
how much you appreciate him. Find ways to please him. Perhaps these actions will give opportunity to take extra steps or
exert extra energy that will burn calories and aid you in
reaching your weight loss goal.

Does he have weaknesses that irritate you? Don't major on
them. Many people have destroyed their marriage by focusing
on negatives. Those who build on faults can expect earth-
quakes in their relationships. Read my book, *Staying Positive
in a Negative World* (Kregel), and apply its teachings to
your marriage. You'll find that you reap what you sow. Love
communicated will come back to you.

Do not allow petty problems or mood swings to keep you
from expressing love. Paul wrote:

> Let the husband render unto the wife due benevo-
> lence: and likewise the wife unto the husband. The
> wife hath not power of her own body, but the hus-
> band: and likewise also the husband hath not power of
> his own body, but the wife. Defraud ye not one the
> other, except it be with consent for a time, that ye
> may give yourselves to fasting and prayer; and come

together again, that Satan tempt you not for your in-
continency (1 Cor. 7:3-5).

This is probably the biblical text husbands and wives neglect most, but it is one of the most powerful to make marriage all it is intended to be. A husband and a wife have
emotional and physical needs, and neither is to hold back in
striving to meet these needs for the other.

Start expressing your love to each other often. This is an
important part of the abundant life God intends you to enjoy.
Both the attitude and the action brought about by an exciting
marriage relationship will help you in all other areas of life.

Especially moving will be the incentive created by this reawakening of your love. That powerful drive may add just the
needed touch to enable you to reach that weight and form
you have desired for so long.

Questions for Application

1. When one or both partners gain weight, how is the marriage affected?

2. How can you and your spouse help each other become
thin, trim, and triumphant? List specific attitudes and actions.

11

The New You

The Christian Diet Class of the Bethany Baptist Church in Mt. Clemens, Michigan began in many years ago. They used *Weight! A Better Way to Lose* as the textbook and my accompanying cassettes as teaching aids. When Doris Zentz, the teacher, wrote me five years later, they were still going strong. She reported that the class had become a large outreach ministry and that during those five years, women from seventy area churches had attended. As I write this chapter, the class continues to thrive.

Why has this outreach been so successful?

One reason is the very capable leadership given the class by Doris Zentz and the present teacher, Dixie Javory. Another is the support of the church. And, of course, the effectiveness of the program cannot be overlooked.

Still another factor that has made this and other similar classes succeed is that each group is ministering to an area of life that has been largely neglected by Bible teachers in churches. In these classes people are learning that God cares about every problem they face and that He wants to give them personal victory, even in the sensitive area of weight control.

This kind of teaching calls for opening up the whole life to the control of the Holy Spirit.

Have you made that kind of surrender?

Others have.

Winning through Surrender

F.B. Meyer, the warmhearted Bible teacher and writer of the past, spoke of a time when he struggled with giving the Lord the keys to all the rooms of his life, especially the key to a small closet that he had reserved for himself. Many of us also forbid the Lord entrance to such private places in our lives. Some reserve the library for themselves, not wanting the Lord to direct their reading. Others prefer to keep Jesus out of the living room, desiring to shut the Lord out of their day to day experiences and submit to Him only on Sunday.[1]

Perhaps you have kept your Lord out of the kitchen or dining room, not considering your diet to be any of His concern. Now you know that He must be Lord of all if you are to enjoy His best.

Henry Varley, a close friend of D.L. Moody in the early days of Moody's ministry, challenged the young evangelist with his now famous statement: "It remains to be seen what God will do with a man who gives himself up wholly to Him." Moody decided that he would be that man, and the world is still reaping the benefits of that decision.

In his book, *Why God Used D.L. Moody*, R. A. Torrey wrote:

> If you and I are to be used in our sphere as D.L. Moody was used in his, we must put all that we have and are in the hands of God, for Him to use as He will, to send us where He will, for God to do with us as He will, and we, on our part, to do everything God bids us do.[2]

"Well," you say, "this is getting rather heavy. I began reading this book because I want to lose weight, and here you are talking about full surrender."

I understand your feelings. But losing weight and developing a lifestyle that keeps you victorious demands your full surrender to Christ. Don't stop short of enjoying God's best every day.

R.A. Torrey explained:

> There are thousands and tens of thousands of men and women in Christian work, brilliant men and women, rarely gifted men and women, men and women who are making great sacrifices, men and women who have put all conscious sin out of their lives, yet who, nevertheless, have stopped short of absolute surrender to God, and therefore have stopped short of the fulness of power. But Mr. Moody did not stop short of absolute surrender to God; he was a wholly surrendered man, and if you and I are to be used, you and I must be wholly surrendered men and women.[3]

The Christian life is the only area in which full surrender brings absolute victory. Absolute victory means triumphant living. And for overweight people, living triumphantly means having the discipline needed to exercise control over food and activity so that desired goals in weight control are achieved.

Abundant life should be the goal of every believer. We should not settle for anything less than God's best. But the full surrender required for abundant living does not come easily for us. Even those who have become well-known for triumphant living have often reached these heights only after periods of spiritual struggle.

The Power of Childlike Faith

J. Hudson Taylor, founder of the China Inland Mission, wrestled with temptation and discouragement that almost drove him to despair. In a letter to his mother, he wrote:

> I cannot tell you how I am buffeted sometimes by

temptation. I never knew how bad a heart I have. Yet I
do know that I love God and love His work, and desire
to serve Him only and in all things. And I value above
all else that precious Saviour in whom alone I can be
accepted. Often I am tempted to think that one so full
of sin cannot be a child of God at all. But I try to
throw it back and rejoice all the more in the precious-
ness of Jesus and in the riches of the grace that has
made us "accepted in the beloved." Beloved, He is of
God; beloved, He ought to be of us. But oh, how short
I fall here again! May God help me love Him more and
serve Him better. Do pray for me. Pray that the Lord
will keep me from sin, will sanctify me wholly, will use
me more largely in His service.[4]

Can this be the great J. Hudson Taylor? Tempted? Having a
bad heart? Thinking himself too full of sin to be a child of God?
Falling short in loving God?

Sounds like you or me.

How many guilt trips have you taken because of your lack of
discipline in eating or carrying through on an exercise program that you had promised yourself you would keep up until
you were thin and trim?

What causes us to lose control to our regret?

There can be but one answer: we battle the same fallen
nature J. Hudson Taylor and other giants of the faith battled
daily.

To be fair to J. Hudson Taylor, however, we need to know
the rest of the story. Six months after he wrote his guilt-
packed letter, a great change took place in Taylor's life. The
change was so great that he declared God had made him a
new man.

What brought about this change? It was a letter from another missionary, John McCarthy.

McCarthy said he had now concluded that striving, longing,
and hoping for better days to come was not the way to holi-
ness, happiness, or usefulness. Instead, he saw that all of these

qualities resided in Christ Himself and that trusting Him completely would provide all he had been seeking.

This simple but powerful truth transformed J. Hudson Taylor's life. As a result, he said he felt as if the dawning of a new and glorious day had risen upon him, adding that he seemed to have reached only the edge of a boundless sea. He now saw in Christ all that he needed to experience power, satisfaction of heart, and unchanging joy. He then wrote:

> How then to have our faith increased? Only by thinking of all that Jesus is and all He is for us: His life, His death, His work, He Himself as revealed to us in the Word, to be the subject of our constant thoughts. Not a striving to have faith ... but looking off to the Faithful One seems all we need; a resting in the Loved One entirely, for time and eternity.[5]

J. Hudson Taylor had been a toiling, burdened Christian with not much rest of soul.

Now he became a bright, happy Christian, experiencing new power and finding new peace. Troubles did not worry him as before. He had traded bondage for liberty and failure for victory. Fear and weakness had been replaced by a restful sense of sufficiency in Christ.

How interesting that such a choice servant of God struggled so long before discovering that the answer he sought was to be found in a moment by moment trust in the Christ who had saved him!

Millions of troubled believers today still miss this seemingly obvious truth.

Taylor had come to experience total trust in all areas of life. Nothing mysterious. Nothing difficult to understand. The great missionary leader had simply learned to trust his Saviour for everything, and this brought him both peace and power.

Childlike faith brings us to the triumphant life. Recognizing this brings every temptation and trial within our power to conquer and every task within the range of accomplishment.

Is This Decision Time?

But it is not enough to know that J. Hudson Taylor learned to live triumphantly. His peace of mind will not remove one wrinkle from *your* troubled brow; his faith will not bring victory over *your* discouragement and depression. His conquest of temptation will not enable *you* to stick with the lifestyle you have chosen to become thin and trim. *You* must trust *your* Saviour daily. Then the triumphant life will become real to you.

Each of the men of faith we have considered came to a time of full surrender of heart and life to Christ.

Have you done the same?

Has a divided heart been keeping you from living triumphantly?

If so, make this your day of new commitment to Christ. Confess your sins to Him and rejoice in His forgiveness. Tell Him you are returning to your first love, and you want only His will for your life.

Share your new commitment to Christ with another person. If you are in a study group, let the entire class know what has happened in your life.

Your new walk with your Saviour will bring many of the thoughts we have shared into proper focus. None of these concepts are difficult to understand. All can be part of your new lifestyle as you walk with Christ in childlike faith.

Surrender and Simplicity

Surrender and *simplicity* are two key words in the triumphant life. Don't try to complicate things that God has made easy to understand.

Evangelist Gypsy Smith was once asked why he always seemed to be in a state of personal revival. "I have never lost the wonder of it all," he replied.

A minister once came to see me because a cloud of depression seemed to hover over him continually. He wondered if life was worth living and asked the Lord many times to end his earthly life and take him to heaven. In his search for answers, he had attended many "deeper life" conferences, and when it was possible, had met alone with the speakers, hoping to find the secret of victory.

As this discouraged man sat across the desk from me, I wondered what I could tell him that had not already been said by another. Then, almost surprised at my own action, I handed him a copy of the Gospel of John and urged him to read it while thinking of himself as one who had just received Christ as his Saviour. I wanted him to return to the basics, refreshing his faith in the simplicity of the Gospel.

This proved to be exactly what this troubled preacher needed.

Beware of those who try to make simple things deep and mysterious. Instead, look for examples in the Bible where deep truths are made simple so that all can understand. Paul told the Christians at Corinth that he wanted them to hold to the simplicity of the Gospel, writing: "But I fear, lest by any means, as the serpent beguiled Eve through his subtilty, so your minds should be corrupted from the simplicity that is in Christ" (2 Cor. 11:3).

What Have You Learned?

Think now how simple the route to becoming thin, trim, and triumphant really is.

God cares about you and is ready to enable you to take off those pounds that you want to lose. His love has been announced in the Bible and proven throughout history. The greatest demonstration of His love is seen in the death of Christ on the cross for us: "But God commendeth His love toward us, in that, while we were yet sinners, Christ died for us" (Rom. 5:8).

It is not wrong to long to be thin as long as your motives do not run counter to any clear teaching of the Bible. You should, however, keep in mind that individuality is important to our Lord, and you should not try to pour yourself into another's mold. Recently, a woman told me that she had to learn that she might never be as thin as she had once hoped to be because that was just not comfortable for her and that it was too difficult to achieve. In her case, I think her decision was sensible and better for her health.

Though there are many different kinds of diets, any diet will work that keeps your intake of calories below what you burn in daily activity. This is so simple that if we are not careful, we will miss it, especially in light of the maze of diets and diet books.

Some lose weight easier than others, due to differences in metabolism. It is not so important that you are losing a great amount weekly or monthly. What is important is establishing a lifestyle that balances eating and exercise so that a *pattern* of losing is established, even though weight may be lost in small amounts. When Elijah prayed for rain, a cloud only the size of a man's hand was enough to convince him that God had answered his prayer. Watch for small victories and make much of them (1 Kings 18:44-46).

Satan is a real enemy who is bent on defeating our efforts to become thin and trim, but we know how to overcome him. As we submit ourselves to God and resist the devil, he will flee from us. Our Lord is greater than this enemy, and provides the strength to win in times of temptation.

Though you have failed at achieving weight control in the past, you can trust the Lord to enable you to succeed this time. And the reason is faith. Shift your confidence from articles in magazines and newspapers about losing weight to the Bible. In childlike faith, accept the truth that God is able to lead you to meaningful weight loss for the sake of your health and the enhancing of your witness for Christ.

Exercise has not been important to you in the past but that is about to change. Refuse to cultivate the art of nonliving. Instead of looking for ways to avoid activity, look for chances to increase your activity in the course of each day.

Decide to stop grieving and quenching the Holy Spirit and walk in the Spirit in simple faith, expecting His control to change your life and make self-control a part of daily experience.

Your marriage was wonderful in those early years and now you know it can be that way again. Determine to do your part by ending selfishness and look for ways to express your love to your husband or wife. Together you'll be able to lose those pounds that threaten your lives and the quality of life.

What a great way to live!

Surrendered to Christ and simply trusting Him each day, you will recapture the warmth of Christian love and living that has escaped you. Determine never again to lose the wonder of it all.

What Is Happening to You?

Something really has begun to happen to you.

You're on your way to becoming thin, trim, and triumphant!

Questions for Application

1. Surrender usually means defeat. How does surrender to Christ bring the victory of abundant living?

2. What does the term childlike faith mean to you? Do you have this kind of faith?

3. Can you think of other heroes of the faith who have experienced periods of spiritual struggle before discovering triumphant living? What can you learn from these men and women?

12

Don't Lose Another Day

Tomorrow I'm going to start my new diet!"

You've heard that line before. Usually it's accompanied by a good-natured laugh while the speaker is downing a banana split or some other high calorie dessert. But taking off extra weight is no laughing matter. Good health and a long life can depend on becoming thin and trim. So if you're overweight, now is the time to begin that new lifestyle that takes off pounds.

Why wait?

Excuses for delay will not remove one unwanted pound and may keep you from ever beginning.

Wise Solomon wrote: "He that observeth the wind shall not sow; and he that regardeth the clouds shall not reap" (Ecc. 11:4).

The Time Is Now

Today is the day to begin.

John Ruskin kept a stone on his desk containing just one word: *Today*. He saw the urgency of seizing the day.

Several years ago I drove across our state to conduct a week of evangelistic services at a country church where I had never been before. Following the pastor's directions that I had received in the mail, I found the church and was immediately impressed. The parking lot was nearly filled. As I approached the front door, I could hear a fine orchestra playing and people singing enthusiastically.

Since I was staying at the parsonage for the week, I had a good opportunity to ask the pastor about his secret of drawing such large crowds to the church in that rural area. I found the answer the first day.

This pastor told me that the three words "Do it now" were key ingredients in his ministry. That very afternoon, he went to visit a member of the church who had been offended by another. He became a peacemaker at once, not allowing that division to go unnoticed and unreconciled. Before nightfall, he had cared for a problem that could have caused trouble in his congregation.

In these chapters we've been sharing a plan for weight control that works. It works because it is based on sound principles and draws its authority and strength from the Book that has answers to all the problems of life—the Bible.

You have no good reason then to delay starting this new lifestyle.

Still some will delay.

Man's nature is to delay even when good will come from moving ahead immediately.

Many delay coming to Christ in faith despite divine assurances that such coming will bring forgiveness and eternal life.

Paul explained:

> We then, as workers together with Him, beseech you also that ye receive not the grace of God in vain. (For he saith, "I have heard thee in a time accepted, and in the day of salvation have I succored thee: behold, now is the accepted time; behold, now is the day of salvation.") (2 Cor. 6:1-2)

One of the most interesting examples of choosing to delay when immediate action would have been better is found in the Book of Exodus and has to do with the plagues that were then falling upon Egypt. The Lord had instructed Moses to tell Pharaoh that unless he allowed the Israelites to leave Egypt, a plague of frogs would come to the land. Pharaoh refused to release the Israelites, and the plague of frogs came upon Egypt as had been promised by the Lord.

Frogs were everywhere in the land. There were frogs in the bedrooms of the people, in their beds, in their kitchens, and even in the kneading troughs where the women were preparing food for their families.

Finally, Pharaoh decided he and his people had suffered enough from this invasion of frogs and called Moses and Aaron before him, supposedly to give in to their demands and to get them to end this plague. The following is the response of Moses to Pharaoh's plea:

> Glory over me: when shall I intreat for thee, and for thy servants, and for thy people, to destroy the frogs from thee and thy houses, that they may remain in the river only? (Ex. 8:9)

Now read Pharaoh's surprising reply:

> And he said, "Tomorrow" (Ex. 8:10).

Pharaoh wanted one more night with the frogs.
Why?
I have no idea.
Neither do I have any idea why anyone would delay adopting a lifestyle that would make it possible for him or her to become thin, trim, and triumphant.
Why do you delay?
Do you enjoy being overweight?
Are you happy about being defeated and depressed?
Recently, I was in a prayer meeting where I heard a woman

ask forgiveness for enjoying her depression.

Can you identify with her?

Do you secretly long to keep on receiving the attention that being overweight brings to you?

The Bondage of Fear

Are you delaying because of fear of failure?

Do you doubt that you will have discipline enough to reduce calories and increase activity? Are you afraid to begin for fear of not carrying through or of losing another battle?

Remember that God understands those anxieties and He cares. Don't miss out on His best for your life by giving in to fear.

When Moses led his people out of Egypt, they were given many assurances of God's protection and provision. The Red Sea opened before them, and they walked through on dry land. Shortly after that, the sea closed upon the armies of Pharaoh who were in hot pursuit.

While on their journey to Canaan, God gave them manna to eat when they were hungry, and fresh cool water from a rock to quench their thirst. A cloud led them by day, and a pillar of fire by night to let them know they were on the route to freedom and the Promised Land.

When they arrived at the border of the land to which they had been traveling, they sent spies into the land to look it over and to report the strength of its inhabitants. What an exciting occasion that must have been for these favored people who had been delivered from slavery and now seemed ready to enter the land that was to become their new home!

Upon the return of the spies, the report of the land's productivity was a glowing one. Everything was as good as had been promised by the Lord. Two of the spies, Joshua and Caleb, urged a quick conquest of the land, but the remaining ten spies spread fear among the people. In their thinking about the coming battles, these doubters disregarded the power of God and saw the opposition as too powerful for them to overcome.

Fear ruled the day.

Instead of advancing in faith as might have been expected after having been miraculously delivered from slavery, they succumbed to fear and fell into depression and regret. Many even called for the appointing of another to replace Moses as their leader. They wanted a captain who would lead them back to Egypt.

How sad!

These delivered slaves could have conquered Canaan through the power of God, but instead they chose to retreat. As a result of their lack of faith, they spent the next forty years wandering in the wilderness. Fear accomplished what the armies of Pharaoh could not do by keeping them from God's best for their lives.

Learn from this tragedy.

Reject fear and move forward in faith.

Triumph in Christ

Adopt this biblical lifestyle that leads to personal joy and victory instead of giving in to fear and continuing in defeat.

You'll find yourself sharing Paul's enthusiasm over the constant triumph that can be ours in every area of life through the power of Christ: "Now thanks be unto God, which always causeth us to triumph in Christ, and maketh manifest the savor of His knowledge by us in every place" (2 Cor. 2:14).

Stop being a victim of obesity when you can be a victor through obedience to the clear teaching of Scripture concerning the abundant life.

Putting It All Together

Remember that God really cares.

Build your faith through a consistent devotional life and through exercising faith daily.

"Submit yourselves therefore to God. Resist the devil, and he will flee from you" (James 4:7).

Stop doubting your ability to reach your goal in weight

control. "For with God nothing shall be impossible" (Luke 1:37).

"Be filled with the Spirit" (Eph. 5:18). By yielding completely to the Holy Spirit, you will receive all the self-control you need because this is part of the fruit of the Spirit, the fruit that makes you thin.

After you have consulted your doctor, embark on a sensible exercise and diet program, looking for opportunities to be more involved in life.

You really can become what you want to be, in the will of God.

But success in weight control begins in beginning.

Don't lose another day.

Question for Application
What will you do today toward your goal of becoming thin, trim, and triumphant? Ask God to help you. Share your plan with someone.

Notes

TWO: IS IT WRONG TO LONG TO BE THIN?

1. Dianne Lawson, "I Almost Starved to Death," *Family Life Today* (Summer, 1984), pp. 25-26.

2. Ibid., p. 28.

3. Arthur Hettich, "Inside our Family Circle," *Family Circle* (Feb. 23, 1988), p. 18.

4. Marie Chapian and Neva Coyle, *There's More to Being Thin Than Being Thin* (Minneapolis: Bethany House Publishers, 1984), p. 124.

5. Carolyn Adams Miller, "Dying to Be Thin," *Family Circle* (Feb. 23, 1988), p. 62.

6. Claudia Wallis, "Gauging the Fat of the Land," *Time* (Feb. 25, 1985), p. 72.

7. William Pauley, "Mr. Before and After," *Power Life*, Scripture Press Publications (April 23, 1967), pp. 4-5.

Organizations Offering Help for Victims of Anorexia Nervosa and Bulimia**

Anorexia Nervosa and Related Eating Disorders, Inc.
P.O. Box 5102
Eugene, OR 97405

Anorexia Nervosa and Related Eating Disorders, Inc.
P.O. Box 7
Highland Park, IL 60035

National Anorexic Aid Society, Inc.
P.O. Box 29461
Columbus, OH 43229

American Anorexia Nervosa Association, Inc.
133 Cedar Lane
Teaneck, NJ 07666

Overeaters Anonymous
Phone (213) 542-8363
Meetings in most states

**If you have symptoms of an eating disorder, contact your doctor immediately.

THREE: WHICH DIET WORKS?

1. Linda Dyett, "A Diet You Can Lose with—and Live with," Your Healthy Body Insert in *Family Circle* (Feb. 2, 1988), pp. 9-10.

2. Laura Stein, "10 Diet Myths," *Ladies Home Journal* (Feb. 1988), p. 163.

3. Dyett, "A Diet You Can Lose with—and Live with," p. 10.

4. Kim Painter, "New Diet for Women Trims Confusion," *USA Today* (Oct. 1, 1986), p. 1.

FOUR: THOSE BORN LOSERS

1. "Prevention's No Diet No Willpower Weight Loss System," *Prevention* (1987), p. 31.

2. Craig Massey, "Pulling through Depression," *Moody Monthly* (April, 1974).

FIVE: THE DEVIL AND YOUR DIET

1. Walter B. Knight, *Three Thousand Illustrations for Christian Service* (Grand Rapids, Michigan: Wm. B. Eerdmans Publishing Company, 1947), pp. 234-235.

2. John R. Rice, *The King of the Jews* (Grand Rapids, Michigan: Zondervan Publishing House), pp. 66-67.

3. Walter B. Knight, *Knight's Treasury of Illustrations* (Grand Rapids, Michigan: Wm. B. Eerdmans Publishing Company, 1963), p. 370.

4. M.R. DeHaan, *Studies in First Corinthians* (Grand Rapids, Michigan: Zondervan Publishing House, 1956), p. 118.

5. Ken Anderson, *Satan's Angels* (Nashville, Tenn.: Thomas Nelson Publishers, 1975), p. 151.

6. Walter B. Knight, *Knight's Treasury of Illustrations*, (Grand Rapids, Michigan: Wm. B. Eerdmans Publishing Company, 1963), p. 422.

SIX: FAITH CAN MOVE THAT MOUNTAIN

1. Charlie Shedd, *The Fat Is in Your Head* (Waco, Texas: Word Books, 1972), pp. 13-14, used by permission.

2. Walter B. Knight, *Knight's Treasury of Illustrations*, (Grand Rapids, Michigan: Wm. B. Eerdmans Publishing Company, 1963), p. 115.

3. Ibid., p. 262.

4. George Müller, "A Narrative of Some of the Lord's dealings with George Müller" *Christianity Today* (March 18, 1988), p. 26.

5. A.W. Tozer, *The Root of the Righteous* (Harrisburg, Penn: Christian Publication, 1955), pp. 49-50.

6. John R. Rice, *Asking and Receiving* (Murfreesboro, Tenn.: Sword of the Lord Publishers, 1942), p. 165.

SEVEN: GET THAT MOUNTAIN MOVING

1. American Society of Bariatric Physicians, "Good, Better, Best Weight-Loss Ideas for 1988," Edited by

Susan Zarrow, *Prevention* (January, 1988), p. 36.

2. Anne Kashiwa and James Rippe, M.D., *Fitness Walking for Women* (New York: Putnam Publishing Group, 1987), p. 75.

3. Ibid., p. 75.

4. Ibid., p. 76.

5. Ibid., p. 74.

EIGHT: THE FRUIT THAT MAKES YOU THIN
    1. Walter B. Knight, *Knight's Master Book of New Illustrations*, (Grand Rapids, Michigan: Wm. B. Eerdmans Publishing Company, 1956), p. 290.

    2. William Pauley, "Mr. Before and After," *Power Life*, Scripture Press Publications (April 23, 1967), p. 5.

ELEVEN: THE NEW YOU
    1. Walter B. Knight, *Knight's Treasury of Illustrations*, (Grand Rapids, Michigan: Wm. B. Eerdmans Publishing Company, 1963), p. 73.

    2. R.A. Torrey, *Why God Used D.L. Moody* (Chicago: The Moody Bible Institute, 1923), p. 10.

    3. Ibid., pp. 10-11.

    4. Dr. and Mrs. Howard Taylor, *Hudson Taylor's Spiritual Secret* (Chicago: Moody Press, 1962), p. 153.

    5. Ibid., p. 156.

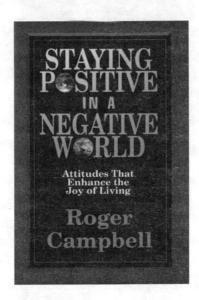

Staying Positive in a Negative World
Attitudes That Enhance the Joy of Living
0-8254-2346-5, 144 pages

"I wrote *Staying Positive in a Negative World* for those who are tired of being down, tired of clouds, tired of valleys," says Roger Campbell. Negativism is a thief, robbing life of adventure and joy. It weakens families, it slows down churches, it kills self-worth. There *is* a better way to live.

That better way begins by knowing that in all circumstances of life, God really cares—and He is at work even in the darkest storms of life. Campbell provides readers with an encouraging guide to spiritual growth.

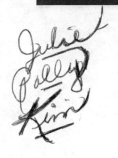

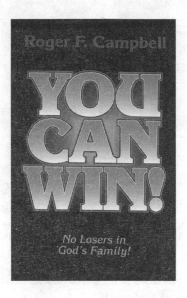

You Can Win!
No Losers in God's Family
0-8254-2323-6, 144 pages

Seasoned author and pastor Roger Campbell calls on believers to use the limitless resources our Lord has provided for spiritual success. Chapter titles include:

"Think Like a Winner"
"Talk Like a Winner"
"Winning Over Temptation"
"Winning Over Worry"

Campbell helps you maintain a positive attitude, lift your sights to higher spiritual goals, and reach for God's best for your life.